HIV/AIDS AS A SECURITY THREAT TO INDIA

The Regional Centre for Strategic Studies (RCSS) is an independent, non-profit and non-governmental organization for collaborative research, networking and interaction on strategic and international issues pertaining to South Asia. Set up in 1992, the RCSS is based in Colombo, Sri Lanka.

The RCSS is a South Asian forum for studies, training and multi-track dialogue and deliberation on issues of regional interest. All activities of RCSS are designed with a South Asia focus and are usually participated by experts from all South Asian countries. The Centre is envisaged as a forum for advancing the cause of co-operation, security, conflict resolution, confidence building, peace and development in the countries of the South Asian region.

The RCSS serves its South Asian and international constituency by: (a) networking programmes that promote interaction, communication and exchange between institutions and individuals within and outside the region engaged in South Asian strategic studies; (b) organizing regional workshops and seminars and sponsoring and coordinating collaborative research-, and (c) disseminating output of the research through publications which include books, monographs and a quarterly newsletter. The RCSS facilitates scholars and other professionals of South Asia to address, mutually and collectively, problems and, issues of topical interest for all countries of the region.

Queries may be addressed to:

Regional Centre for Strategic Studies
2 Elibank Road
Colombo 5
SRI LANKA
Tel: (94-11) 2599734, 2599735
Fax: 2599993; e-mail: edrcss@sri.lanka.net
RCSS website: http://www.rcss.org

RCSS Policy Studies 28

HIV/AIDS as a Security Threat to India

HAPPYMON JACOB

REGIONAL CENTRE FOR STRATEGIC STUDIES
COLOMBO

MANOHAR
2005

Published by
Ajay Kumar Jain for
Manohar Publishers & Distributors
4753/23 Ansari Road, Daryaganj
New Delhi 110 002
and
Regional Centre for Strategic Studies
2 Elibank Road
Colombo 5
SRI LANKA
Tel: (94-11) 2599734-5; Fax: 2599993;
e-mail: edrcss@sri.lanka.net
website: http://www.rcss.org

First published 2005

ISBN 81-7304-630-1

Printed at
Lordson Publishers Pvt Ltd
Delhi 110 007

Distributed in South Asia by
FOUNDATION BOOKS
4381/4, Ansari Road
Daryaganj, New Delhi 110 002
and its branches at Mumbai, Hyderabad,
Bangalore, Chennai, Kolkata

Contents

Acknowledgements 7

Introduction 9

1. HIV/AIDS in India: An Overview 13
   - HIV/AIDS in India: History, Status and Future 13
   - The Future of AIDS in India 29
   - Conclusion 34
2. HIV/AIDS as a Threat to Security 35
   - HIV/AIDS as a Traditional Security Threat 35
   - HIV/AIDS as a Human Security Threat 41
   - HIV/AIDS as an Economic Security Threat 44
   - Setbacks in the Global Market Place? 51
   - HIV/AIDS as a Societal Security Threat 60
   - Conclusion 65
3. Three Dangerous Factors: Poverty, Ignorance and Stigma 67
   - Poverty and AIDS 67
   - Ignorance and AIDS 69
   - Stigma and AIDS 72
   - Conclusion 74
4. The Experiences of Other Regions/Countries 76
   - HIV/AIDS: The African Experience 76
   - South Africa: The Triumph of HIV/AIDS 78
   - Thailand's Success Story 82
   - Conclusion 84
5. Conclusion: Where are We Heading? 85

Bibliography 91

RCSS is grateful to the
Ford Foundation for its generous
support for the Kodikara Award
on which this report is based.

Acknowledgements

Prof. Sridhar Khatri has been largely responsible for the successful completion of this work, not only because the Regional Centre for Strategic Studies (RCSS), of which he is the director, supported me financially to conduct the study, but more so because he was a constant source of motivation during the course of this study. I am grateful to him for the gentle but firm reminders, sound advice, and consistent encouragement.

I will always be indebted to Prof. Kanti Bajpai for his lessons on conceptual clarity, methodological rigour and the insights on the non-traditional security discourse. He was a constant source of inspiration from the time I applied for the Kodikara Award until the time I submitted the final product to the RCSS.

Being a wonderful human being, Prof. Amitabh Mattoo is also a great guru who understands the Confucian maxim, 'Give a person a fish and you feed him for a day; teach a person to fish and you feed him for a lifetime.' I am indebted to him for all his friendly advice and academic encouragement.

I am also indebted to Ambassador Teresita C. Schaffer for her many immensely useful suggestions. She made me aware of the importance of the topic I was working on even though my interactions with her were very few.

I would also like to express my deep sense of gratitude to the large number of doctors, health workers, NGO workers and, most importantly, sex workers whom I interacted with all over India during my field survey. Without their support this study would not have happened.

HAPPYMON JACOB

Introduction

The basic proposition of this paper is that HIV/AIDS is a security threat to India. Security may be understood as a state of being secure from threats. However, security is not a monolithic concept; it has many constituent parts, which need not be confined to a predefined number. Barry Buzan, in *People, States and Fear*, spells out five such parts, or 'sections' as he calls them, of security: military, political, economic, societal and environmental.[1] What is strikingly new about his argument is that by way of sectioning security, he is fundamentally challenging the singular approach to traditional security studies whose sole focus is military security. Buzan also takes issue with traditional security studies saying that individuals are as important as the state, 'The security of individuals is locked into an unbreakable paradox in which it is partly dependent on and partly threatened by the state.'[2]

Barry Buzan's critique is an extension of the realist project with a critical turn. Thus, it does not go all out to reject and restructure the 'referent object' of traditional security studies—the security of the state. Ken Booth's path-breaking article titled 'Security and Emancipation' takes on this critical distancing from the state. For Booth, 'individuals are the ultimate referent objects of security.'[3] He also argues that emancipation of the individual is his/her security. David Mutimer further explains what Booth means when he speaks of emancipation:

[1] Barry Buzan, *People, States and Fear: An Agenda for International Security Studies in the Post-Cold War Era*, Boulder, 1991, p. 19.

[2] Ibid., p. 364.

[3] Ken Booth, 'Security and Emancipation', *Review of International Studies*, vol. 17, 1991, p. 319.

Because security aims to 'protect' a referent object from threat, it will tend to privilege the present condition of that referent. To make the state or a society the referent object of security is to privilege its continued existence in its present form. One of the striking features of Booth's reformulation of security in terms of emancipation is that it turns this conservatism on its head.[4]

The question here is, who does HIV/AIDS threaten? Does it threaten the 'state', the military, the individual, the society, as the Copenhagen school would have it, or is it something else? Having looked at HIV/AIDS and its pace of growth and potential for destruction, I consider that HIV/AIDS is not a single referent-object-threat; rather, it threatens the security of many sectors of the nation, the individual being only one of them.

Increasingly, the state is being understood not as a monolithic entity but as something that is made up of many constituent parts or sectors. A state is not necessarily a given or eternal; it is a dynamic whole constituted by many parts which inhere in the former. With such an understanding of the state, it would be inappropriate to privilege one sector over another. What also needs to be understood is that since all threats are not of similar nature, sectors which may be affected or threatened will not be the same in the case of each and every threat. Therefore, one need not prejudge the sector or sectors in a conception of security; sectorizing security should be done only after measuring the level of insecurity from a threat perception.

What is the referent object in security—the state or something else? This question assumes notions like 'there should be 'one' referent object in the conception of security', and 'this referent object has to be predetermined'. I would disagree with both notions. There need not be one referent object in the security conception all the time. So the answer to the question 'security for whom?' would be 'security for that which is threatened.' Secondly, we need not predetermine which referent object should be the most important one in analyzing a particular threat to

[4] David Mutimer, 'Beyond Strategy', in Craig A. Snyder (ed.), *Contemporary Security and Strategy*, London: Macmillan, 1999, p. 86.

security, as mentioned earlier. The referent object of security is the object of threat at a specifically given point of time. The referent object/s has/have to be conceived as a dynamic entity/ies and not as predetermined and/or stagnant.

What is the 'ultimate' referent object of security? Shouldn't there be a referent object beyond all these peripherally constituted referent objects like society, military, economy, etc.? Not necessarily. There is no such abstracted notion of a human being that has to be venerated as the ultimate referent object of security, nor should we necessarily see the universe as anthropocentric. Human beings are not abstract stand alone entities but constructions of so many factors which are equally important. Security, therefore, has to be seen and understood not as single-entity-centric, but as multiple-entity-centric.

Finally, I do not accept Ole Waever's advice on desecuritizing issues so that we don't end up having militarized solutions, because, as Mutimer rightly says: 'by desecuritising issues we are privileging, in some ways, some issues to be securitised with its attendant attention and subsequent material resources.'[5] Ole Waever's argument assumes that security is primarily about militarized issues, which has come under a lot of criticism in the recent literature on security studies. Moreover, as James Der Derian points out, 'No other concept in international relations packs the metaphysical punch, nor commands the disciplinary power of security.... And, less often noted in international relations, in its name billions have been made and millions killed while scientific knowledge has been furthered and intellectual dissent muted.'[6]

HIV/AIDS is a security threat to India because it threatens the economic, human, societal, and even the traditional notions of security. This paper seeks to build up this argument with an understanding of security as spelt out in the preceding paragraphs and see how these various sectors of India's security are threatened by HIV/AIDS.

[5] Mutimer, 'Beyond Strategy', p. 97.

[6] James Der Derian, 'The Value of Security: Hobbes, Marx, Nietzsche, and Baudrillard,' in Ronnie Lipschutz (ed.), *On Security*, New York: Columbia University Press, 1995, pp. 24–5.

The first chapter gives an overview of India's HIV/AIDS epidemic; its history and current status, and also takes a brief look at the future of AIDS in India. The second chapter looks at how the disease is a traditional, human, economic, and societal security issue. The third chapter will analyze three dangerous scenarios for India *vis-à-vis* HIV/AIDS. This chapter will look at how poverty, ignorance, and social stigma regarding HIV/AIDS along with the disease itself can prove to be disastrous for India's security. The final chapter will look at the HIV/AIDS situation in sub-Saharan Africa. This section will highlight the fact that the spread of HIV/AIDS in Africa, including South Africa, has much in common with India, and learning from their experiences and contrasting them with the Thai experience would be instructive.

CHAPTER 1

HIV/AIDS in India: An Overview

This chapter takes a brief look at the history, status, and the future of HIV/AIDS in India. It addresses a range of issues such as the various estimates of the infection in the country provided by the Government of India (and those who criticize it and quote alternative figures), the extent of the disease in different states, the steady spread of the epidemic to the interior regions and the general public, the ways in which the disease is spreading, and how the various factors are making the epidemic assume dangerous proportions.

The chapter begins with an examination of the various estimates about the working-age population in India and how they can be affected by the HIV/AIDS threatening the country's economic security. The sections that follow look at the history and status of the epidemic in the country. The chapter concludes with a section on the future of AIDS in India.

HIV/AIDS IN INDIA: HISTORY, STATUS AND FUTURE

The working-age population in India will see an unprecedented increase in the next 20–30 years; in 2001, 62.1 per cent of India's population was estimated to be in the working-age group, and is expected to be 64.2 in 2021, and 63.6 in 2031, followed by a decline thereafter.[1] This increase in the working-age population of the country is significant for three reasons. First, for many

[1] While the UN considers those who fall between the ages of 15 and 59 as the working-age population, the International Labour Organisation (ILO) considers those between the ages of 15 and 64 as belonging to the working-age population.

countries like the US, China and Japan, this surge in the working-age population is over. Second, for India, this is an unprecedented increase in the working-age population. Third, the Indian economy is in a stage of receiving the economic benefits of economic globalization and this is fortunately coinciding with the increase in the working-age population (see Table 1.1).

There is, however, going to be a setback. If the working-age of the population is going to be a key factor in India's economic growth in the years to come, it is precisely this group that is afflicted by the wide and rapid spread of HIV/AIDS.

Nicholas Eberstadt has provided a depressing picture of India's working-age population under three scenarios *vis-à-vis* HIV/AIDS.[2]

Economy is just one aspect of a country's security that is adversely affected by HIV/AIDS. There are other important aspects like human security, societal security, and even traditional notions of security that are increasingly jeopardized by HIV/AIDS.

While there has been a reluctance among Indian scholars, both those who study national security and those who look at its social and economic underpinnings, to link security and HIV/AIDS, many leading think tanks already consider it a security issue. America's Central Intelligence Agency (CIA) added HIV/AIDS incidence to the list of variables that should be considered when analysing which states were likely to be unstable or collapse in the

TABLE 1.1: WORKING-AGE POPULATION IN 2025

	Without HIV	Mild Epidemic	Intermediate Epidemic	Severe Epidemic
China	1.0 billion	981 million	963 million	947 million
India	932 million	910 million	879 million	854 million
Russia	89 million	86 million	81 million	78 million

Source: Nicholas Eberstadt.

[2] Nicholas Eberstadt, 'The Future of AIDS', *Foreign Affairs,* vol. 81, no. 6, November/December 2002, p. 37.

future.[3] US assessments express concern about the rising problem of HIV/AIDS by 2010 in five countries of strategic importance to the US that have large populations at risk for HIV-infection: Nigeria, Ethiopia, Russia, India, and China.[4] The International Crisis Group has termed it as a personal, economic, communal, national, and international security issue.[5] An *Adelphi Paper* published by the International Institute of Strategic Studies (IISS) reasons that 'pending a cure and vaccine, it would be a very risky social and strategic experiment simply to let HIV/AIDS rage in strategically significant countries like China, India and Russia.'[6]

A report published by the Centre for Strategic and International Studies, Washington, says that 'HIV/AIDS is now recognized as a major threat to India's health and economy by elites throughout the country. Indian NGOs have done much to raise the visibility of AIDS in the country.'[7] The UN also has recognized the importance of this threat. During the first session of the UNSC in 2000, HIV/AIDS was declared to be a major threat to international security.

If a country has 1 per cent of its population infected with HIV/AIDS, it is considered to be an epidemic. Moreover, if more than 5 per cent of the adult population is infected, health officials say, it is difficult to keep the disease from accelerating. Almost 1 per cent of India's present population is infected. While it is true that there is a difference of 4 per cent between 1 per cent and

[3] Stefan Elbe, 'Strategic implications of HIV/AIDS', *Adelphi Paper*, no. 357, The International Institute for Strategic Studies, 2003.

[4] David F. Gorden, 'The Next Wave of HIV/AIDS: Nigeria, Ethiopia, Russia, India, and China', US Intelligence Community Assessment, p. 1, September 2002, available at www.cia.gov/nic/PDF_GIF_otherprod/ HIVAIDS/ICA_HIVAIDS20092302.pdf.

[5] 'HIV/AIDS as a Security Issue', International Crisis Group, 19 June 2001, available at http://www.crisisweb.org//library/documents/report_archive/A400321_19062001.pdf.

[6] Elbe, 'Strategic implications of HIV/AIDS', p. 65.

[7] Teresita C. Schaffer and Pramit Mitra, 'India at the Crossroads: Confronting the HIV/AIDS Challenge, A Report of the CSIS HIV/AIDS Delegation to India', 3–10 January 2004, p. 10, available at www.csis.org/saprog/0401_hivindia.pdf.

5 per cent, the huge numbers infected by HIV/AIDS in the 1 billion plus population of India is a massive problem. In this context it may be recalled that a decade ago, South Africa had a prevalence rate of only 1 per cent, whereas today it officially has the largest number of people living with HIV/AIDS.[8] The Chief of UNAIDS, Dr Peter Piot, thinks that there is every possibility that India may overtake South Africa in the number of AIDS cases in just a few years time.[9] In 2001, South Africa had 20.1 per cent of its population infected with HIV/AIDS, which is an estimated 13 per cent of the world's total HIV/AIDS-infected population, and going by the antenatal test results of 2002, the prevalence rate was 26.5 per cent in 2002.[10]

The world's first AIDS case was reported in June 1981. Since then more than 25 million people have died of AIDS the world over. India's first anti-HIV antibodies were detected in Chennai in 1986, followed by the first case of AIDS in India in Mumbai in the same year.[11]

While India's HIV/AIDS infection rate has not reached the important 1 per cent mark among the general population, some Indian cities and regions are already reporting infection rates of more than 5 per cent.[12] For example, 2 or more per cent of pregnant women in Mumbai are reportedly HIV-positive, and the percentage is shooting up to five in parts of Tamil Nadu.[13] The 2003 estimates by the National AIDS Control Organisation of India (NACO) reported that there were 4.58 million Indians living with HIV/AIDS in 2002. It also mentioned that there were 6,10,000 new infections in 2002.[14] While these numbers are often

[8] Elbe, 'Strategic Implications of HIV/AIDS', pp. 16-17.

[9] 'UN Says India May Overtake South Africa in AIDS Cases', 5 June 2002, available at http://www.hivandhepatitis.com/recent/developing/050602f.html.

[10] 'HIV/AIDS in South Africa', 10 August 2004, available at http://www.avert.org/aidssouthafrica.htm

[11] Dr. Nitin Shah, 'HIV/AIDS', available at http://www.medivisionindia.com/aids/index.phtml.

[12] 'HIV/AIDS as a Security Issue', International Crisis Group report, p. 3, available at www.crisisweb.org/home/getfile.cfm?id=510&type=pdf.

[13] Ibid., p. 8.

[14] These estimates were given by the National AIDS Control Organisation, available at http://www.naco.nic.in/indianscene/esthiv.htm.

laughed off, a brief look at the figures of past years can shed new light on the spread of this disease.

In 1986, the number of people who were infected with the HIV virus in India was two. Seventeen years later, in 2003, the figure stood at 5.1 million. The figures were 3.5, 3.7, 3.86, 3.97, 4.58 and 5.1 million, respectively, in 1998, 1999, 2000, 2001, 2002, and 2003. Table 1.2 gives the figures for HIV/AIDS for various years.

TABLE 1.2: PEOPLE LIVING WITH HIV/AIDS, 1986-2002

1986	2
1990	2,00,000
1994	17,50,000
1998	35,00,000
1999	37,00,000
2000	38,60,000
2001	39,70,000
2002	45,80,000

Source: National AIDS Control Organisation. [15]

Even if one is to go strictly by what the government officials say, the future scenario is no better. A CSIS HIV/AIDS delegation to India quotes Meenakshi Dutta Ghosh, Director of the National AIDS Control Organisation (NACO), as having said in late 2002 that even 'if NACO met its programme goals, HIV-infection would grow to 9 million by 2010; if it fell short of its goals by 50 per cent, infections would rise to 14.7 million'.[16] Going by the success rates of the Indian government's action plans in other fields, one would be justified in suspecting that there would be at least 15 million infections by 2010. In 2004, the World Bank said in a report on HIV/AIDS in India that if there is no substantial change in the treatment policy and progress on prevention, HIV/AIDS will become the single largest cause of death in India by 2033 with the disease accounting for 17 per cent of all deaths and

[15] See website of the National AIDS Control Organisation, India, www.naco.org.

[16] Teresita C. Schaffer et al., 'India at the Crossroads', p. 6.

40 per cent of infectious deaths (at present it accounts for 2 per cent of all deaths and 6 per cent of infectious deaths). The report further said that if no urgent further steps are taken to stop the spread of the disease, 'the number of Indians contracting AIDS could rise to 5.5 million a year by 2033.'[17] Tables 1.3, 1.4 and 1.5 describe the future scenarios of HIV/AIDS in India as laid out by Eberstadt.

TABLE 1.3: CUMULATIVE NEW HIV CASES IN 2000–2025

	Mild Epidemic	Intermediate Epidemic	Severe Epidemic
China	32 million	70 million	100 million
India	30 million	110 million	140 million
Russia	4 million	13 million	19 million

Source: Eberstadt.[18]

TABLE 1.4: POPULATION IN 2025

	Without HIV	Mild Epidemic	Intermediate Epidemic	Severe Epidemic
China	1.46 billion	1.42 billion	1.39 billion	1.37 billion
India	1.38 billion	1.34 billion	1.30 billion	1.26 billion
Russia	0.14 billion	0.13 billion	0.12 billion	0.12 billion

Source: Eberstadt.[19]

Government figures have been repudiated by most health and social workers across the country as well as external agencies. There are, in fact, many problems in the way the Government of India takes stock of the HIV/AIDS situation in the country. First, let us take a look at the way these figures are arrived at by .NACO. NACO uses sentinel surveillance data collected from women attending antenatal clinics, STD clinic attendees, injecting drug

[17] 'India faces explosion in HIV/AIDS', 14 August 2004, available at http://www.guardian.co.uk/india/story/0,12559,1282852,00.html.

[18] Eberstadt, 'The Future of AIDS', p. 35.

[19] Ibid., p. 37.

TABLE 1.5: NEW AIDS CASES IN 2015

	Mild Epidemic	Intermediate Epidemic	Severe Epidemic
China	1.2 million	2.6 million	3.9 million
India	1.0 million	3.0 million	4.9 million
Russia	0.2 million	0.5 million	0.7 million

Source: Eberstadt.[20]

users and men having sex with men. As of 2001, a total of 237 select sites were used for this purpose from all over the country, of which there were 109 STD clinics, 110 clinics for pregnant women, 11 sites for injecting drug users, and 2 for men having sex with men. Indrani Gupta et al., rightly say that full-blown

AIDS cases were not included at the time of calculating the estimates using sentinel surveillance data, and the age range in focus was 15-49 years. Also, sex workers are not currently being included as a sentinel group in the surveillance. Lack of adequate representation of all the risk groups (including those not traditionally regarded as high risk groups) as well as lack of proper geographic spread—including proper representation from rural areas—in sentinel surveillance, clearly highlight the need for involving these subpopulations and non-government organizations having active contact with some of the 'hard to reach population' such as IDUs and MSMs in surveillance activities.[21]

This shows the lacunae in arriving at the current figures. Moreover, HIV/AIDS surveillance in India is based purely on urban government hospitals. Private hospitals, which cater to around 80 per cent of health care in the country, are also not taken into account. What should also be taken into account is the allegation

[20] Ibid., p. 36.

[21] Indrani Gupta, Samiran Panda and Renuka Motihar, 'HIV/AIDS and Development in India', Background Study for the Swedish Country Strategy for India 2003–7, February 2003, p. 14, available at http://www.countryanalyticwork.net/CAW/Cawdoclib.nsf/vewWhatsnewLatestDocument/33E1C61C8AE8E58885256E31004D8FF6/$file/HIV-AIDSDevIndia03.pdf.

that most Indian laboratories do not stick to the internationally accepted quality standards for HIV testing.[22]

That is why there is, in fact, a huge difference between the official figures and those arrived at by others both in India and elsewhere. The US National Intelligence Council (USNIC) report says that the number was between 5 and 8 million people in 2002. In 2002, USNIC estimated that by 2025 India would have 20–25 million people affected by HIV/AIDS. The same report predicted that by the same year China would have only 10–15 million cases.[23]

Dr Ishwar Gilada of the Mumbai-based People's Health Organisation, opines that 'currently it is doubling at the rate of 18 months, or at the rate of every 24 months. And I am estimating something like 10 to 12 million HIV-infections today.'[24]

Dr Subhash Hira, Director of the AIDS Research and Control Centre, Mumbai, says that his organization's 'surveillance centres have reported about 38 lakh patients with HIV/AIDS all over the country in December 2000. By 2004, this could rise to 80 lakhs or 1 crore. In Mumbai today, four out of five cases showing symptoms of possible AIDS-related infections, turn out to be so.'[25] In 2003, the United Nations Development Programme (UNDP) predicted that India is likely to have 110 million cases of HIV/AIDS by the year 2025, and this would, the report says, mean an estimated reduction of life expectancy by 13 years.[26] Dr Suniti Solomon, Director of the Tamil Nadu-based YRG Care, says, 'not

[22] Maria Ekstrand, Lisa Garbus and Elliot Marseille, 'HIV/AIDS in India', AIDS Policy Research Center, University of California San Francisco, August 2003, p. 6, available at http://ari.ucsf.edu/ARI/policy/profiles/India.pdf.

[23] Gorden, 'The Next Wave of HIV/AIDS: Nigeria, Ethiopia, Russia, India, and China.'

[24] 'AIDS in India', 26 June 2001, online interview appeared in *The NewsHour*, available from http://www.pbs.org/newshour/bb/health/jan-june01/aidsindia_6-26.html.

[25] 'One crore Indians may be affected by AIDS', *Times of India*, New Delhi, 13 May 2001.

[26] 'India to have 110 million HIV/AIDS victims by 2025', 25 August 2004, available at http://www.newindpress.com/Newsitems.asp?ID=IEH20030708132100&Title=Top+Stories&rLink=0.

so long ago I would perhaps see one HIV/AIDS patient in a week—now it is more like eight a day.'[27]

Dr Rajan Gupta, a nuclear physicist at the Los Alamos National Laboratory in the US, who has written extensively on the HIV/AIDS situation in India, says that there will be 50 million infections in 2007 and 100 million by 2010. This is overwhelming because it would mean roughly, as he says, 'one in ten people, i.e. on average of one in every family. Also, it is important to realize that all socio-economic levels are already affected. Thus life as we know of will cease to exist by year 2010, if not sooner.'[28]

Given the huge disparity between the figures provided by different agencies, both internal and external, it is possible for many to discount whistle-blowers and those who come out with the higher numbers. It is important that such sceptics remember that, in 1989, leading epidemiologists had predicted that there would be 2–3 million people living with AIDS by 1996 the world over: in 1996, there were, in fact, 10.4 million people living with AIDS.[29]

One of the biggest problems with HIV/AIDS is that since there is a huge gap between the time of HIV infection and the time of falling prey to AIDS, many people today are unaware of their HIV status. Moreover, since tuberculosis (TB) is the most likely infection in those who are HIV-positive, many are likely to mistake AIDS for TB, forgetting that almost 30 per cent of people with HIV are also infected with TB.[30]

Indian states are divided into three categories based on the rate of prevalence in each of them. Group A states are called the high-prevalent or generalized epidemic states, which include Maharashtra, Tamil Nadu, Karnataka, Andhra Pradesh (AP), Manipur, and

[27] Subhadra Menon, 'India's Widening AIDS Epidemic', BBC News, 28 November 2003, available at http://news.bbc.co.uk/2/hi/south_asia/3250285.stm.

[28] Deepal Jayasekera, 'AIDS becomes a serious health problem in India', 4 May 2001, available at http://www.wsws.org/articles/2001/may2001/aids-m04.shtml.

[29] 'HIV/AIDS as a Security Issue', ICG Report, p. 1.

[30] 'The HIV/AIDS crisis in India', *South Asia Monitor*, Centre for Strategic and International Studies, 1 May 2003, available at http://www.csis.org/saprog/sam58.pdf.

Nagaland. In these states the HIV-infection rate has crossed the crucial 1 per cent level or more in antenatal women. Group B states (moderate-prevalent or concentrated HIV-epidemic states) are those states where the HIV-infection has reached 5 per cent or more among high-risk groups but the infection is below 1 per cent among antenatal women. Gujarat, Goa, Pondicherry, Mizoram and West Bengal fall in this category. All the remaining states and Union Territories are in the third category, that is, low HIV-epidemic or low-prevalent states where the infection is less than 5 per cent in all high-risk groups, and less than 1 per cent in antenatal women.

The high-prevalent states have been infected by HIV/AIDS in two ways. While Maharashtra, Karnataka and Andhra Pradesh are victims of migration and AIDS spread through sex workers and truck drivers, the north-eastern states have been affected by intravenous drug use.[31]

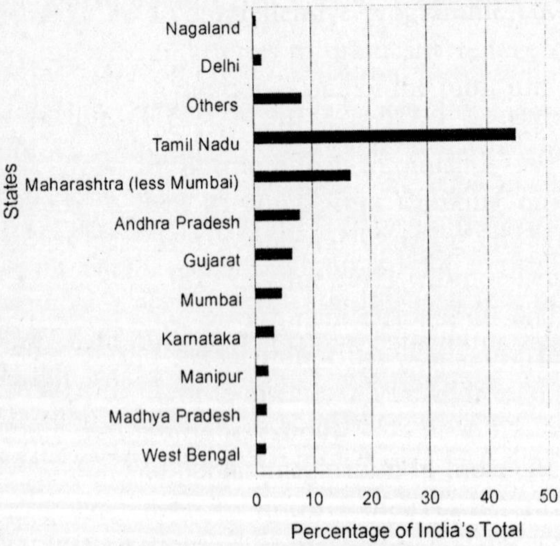

Source: National AIDS Control Organisation.[32]

FIGURE 1.1: DISTRIBUTION OF AIDS CASES BY STATE THROUGH AUGUST 2003

[31] 'The HIV/AIDS Crisis in India', CSIS, 1 May 2003, p. 7.

[32] National AIDS Control Organisation, India.

While it was traditionally thought that HIV/AIDS infects the high-risk groups and spreads in certain pockets of high-prevalent states, to say that today would amount to sheer ignorance. It is widely acknowledged today that HIV is spreading to rural areas through migrant workers and truck drivers. Surveys show that 5–10 per cent of truck drivers in the country are infected with HIV/AIDS, and they pass it on to far-flung villages of the country.[33] It is no exaggeration to say that the general public has become the high-risk population today. Sex workers, truckers, migrant labour, prisoners, troops stationed in remote areas are all part of the 'high-risk group' today.[34] If we add to this the family members of all these people, we are talking about huge chunks of India's population who do not necessarily live in high-prevalent states, but could live anywhere in the country including remote villages. In fact, apart from these usual high-risk groups, fishermen, housewives, office-goers, IT professionals, students, street children, slum dwellers, and blood donors also belong to the 'high-risk' group.

Almost all the doctors and health workers this author spoke with in cities like Mumbai, Chennai, Bangalore, Hyderabad, Pune, and Delhi say that newer areas are reporting HIV/AIDS cases. In fact, Dr Meenakshi Dutta Ghosh stated in July 2003 that HIV/AIDS is no longer affecting only high-risk groups or urban populations, but 'is gradually spreading into rural areas and the general population.'[35] In fact, today 51 per cent of those infected with HIV/AIDS in India are residents of rural India.[36] The situation is getting out of control in the worst hit states. *The Indian Express* reported on 15 September 2004 that during random checks on pregnant woman visiting prenatal clinics in Vijayawada city, over 10 per cent of them tested positive for the deadly virus.

[33] 'HIV/AIDS in India', available at http://www.genetics.wayne.edu/asg/hivindia.html.

[34] Schaffer et al., 'India at the Crossroads', p. 7.

[35] Ekstrand et al., 'HIV/AIDS in India', p. 19.

[36] 'Growth of AIDS in India declines', *The New Delhi Television*, 6 July 2004, New Delhi, available at http://www.ndtv.com/template/template.asp?id=56707&template=AIDS&callid=1&frmsrch=1&txtsrch=hiv%2Faids.

For example, Delhi is not considered to be a high-risk state. In 2001, *The Pioneer* reported that 'one per cent of all the pregnant women in the capital are HIV-positive with chances that 30 per cent of the children from these births would get infected with the virus'.[37] The newspaper was quoting the figures released by the Indian Academy of Pediatrics. An NGO called CHELSEA, which is implementing HIV intervention programmes in a slum area with a population of more than a lakh within a general community location in East Delhi, came across 92 HIV-positive cases after having worked in the locality for merely five months.[38]

When a medical camp was conducted in a school in Madurai, 7 students in the age group of 14 to 18 tested HIV-positive. The same report also said that a professional college near Madurai too had a similar experience, where at least 16 students of the college were tested positive for HIV in a similar camp.[39] The myth that HIV/AIDS is a 'city sickness' is also getting shattered with survey results proving the contrary often enough. A survey of selected households in Tamil Nadu by a team led by Dr Suniti Solomon found that 2.1 per cent of the adult population living in the countryside was HIV-infected compared with 0.7 per cent of the urban population.[40]

Cedric Fernandez of the Sahara Foundation, Pune, who this author talked to in Pune, testified that the infection is rapidly spreading to villages. He claims that his dispensary in the outskirts of Pune gets HIV patients from all walks of life and all parts of the state. George Swamy of the John Paul Slum Development Trust also confirmed to this author that the disease is spreading to

[37] '1 per cent of pregnant women are HIV positive', *The Pioneer*, New Delhi, 2 November 2001.

[38] Mail sent by Dr Ashok Agarwal, Technical Advisor – HIV/AIDS, Catholic Relief Services, Kolkata, India to Yahoo AIDS India Forum in 2002.

[39] '7 Madurai School kids test HIV-positive', *Indian Express*, New Delhi, 31 January 2003.

[40] Suniti Solomon and Aylur Kailasm Ganesh, 'HIV in India', International AIDS Society–USA, *Topics in HIV Medicine*, vol. 10, no. 3, July/August 2002, p. 20, available at http://www.iasusa.org/pub/topics/2002/issue3/july_august 2002.pdf.

the far-flung villages of Maharashtra. Aditya Bandophadyaya told this author in Hyderabad that it would therefore be a huge mistake not to concentrate on villages but only on cities.[41]

Reports do suggest that various towns of Uttar Pradesh (UP), which is a low-prevalent state, like Lucknow, Faizabad, Rae Bareli, Basti, and Gorakhpur record a high number of HIV/AIDS cases.[42] A senior faculty member at the King George Medical College (KGMC) in UP says that unreported cases in the state are at least 10 times higher.[43] The state has a population of around 170 million and is one of the least progressive states in literacy, governance, and economic development. Schaffer et al., point out that '[s]everal major national highways pass through this state. Data from antenatal clinics come only from 17 of the state's 70 districts.'[44] Ms Namrata Chauhan, Mental Health Professional and Consultant in HIV/AIDS and disability related issues based in UP, says that the mapping of HIV/AIDS in the state is in no way considered to be good because it keeps the figures low. Moreover, the state has a large migrant population which is increasingly spreading the disease to the villages in the state.[45] All this shows that it will not be very long before UP becomes a high-prevalent state.

In Bihar, Jharkhand, Chhattisgarh and Orissa, again low-prevalent states, the number of HIV/AIDS infected persons is growing due to the large number of people (from these states) who work as labourers or domestic help in the country's metropolitan centres. Statistics presented in a seminar (conducted in Ranchi) on 'Trafficking and Immigration in Jharkhand' brought to light the fact that 76,000 female labourers in Delhi, 55,000 in Kolkata,

[41] Interviews with Cedric Fernandez and Goerge Swamy in Pune on 13 February 2004. Interview with Aditya Bandophadyaya of *Mitroodu* (A group for the HIV-infected homosexuals) in Hyderabad on 8 February 2004.

[42] 'Number of HIV-infected women growing in UP', *Times of India*, New Delhi, 28 March 2001.

[43] Ibid.

[44] Schaffer et al., 'India at the Crossroads', p. 17.

[45] Namrata Chauhan, Honorary Consultant, AIDS Awareness Centre for Counselling Education and Training (AACCET), Isabella Thoburn College, Faizabad Road, Lucknow. Personal email communication with the author in March 2004.

35,000 in Mumbai, and 13,000 in Chennai belonged to Jharkhand, Orissa, and Chhattisgarh.[46] The chances are very high that these women will get infected with HIV/AIDS and bring it back to their families, infecting both the 'no-AIDS' states and the remote villages.

Bihar's health officials say that the state is showing a disturbing increase in HIV/AIDS infections with migrant labourers and truck drivers being the major vectors of the disease.[47] However, the State AIDS Control Society failed to identify even a single person suffering from AIDS or carrying HIV among the high-risk groups through non-governmental organizations during 1999–2001, although the target was 1,13,500 persons. The AIDS Control Society could only open two licensed blood banks in the district hospitals against a target of five. The society could also not supply any medicine to the AIDS patients admitted in the different medical college hospitals of the state.[48] While talking to this author in Chennai, Dr Jaya Shreedhar mentioned that many states, including Bihar, were not utilizing even the funds allocated to them for the prevention and care of HIV/AIDS victims, leave alone asking for more funds.[49] A Muzaffarpur-based NGO said that at least 40 cases of HIV/AIDS are detected by the organization every month. Doctors at the Patna-based Sen Diagnostics said that from October 2001 to March 2002, the centre tested 474 samples, of which 97 were positive.[50]

Other low-prevalent states are not far behind in this race to get into the top group. *The Telegraph* reported in 2001 that two new HIV-positive persons on an average every day are coming to the

[46] Pawanpreet Singh, '30 labourers return with AIDS', *Times of India*, New Delhi, 20 March 2004.

[47] 'Alarming increase in HIV/AIDS cases in Bihar', *Hindustan Times*, New Delhi, 9 March 2002.

[48] 'AIDS control program in Bihar a total failure', *Times of India*, 15 July 2001.

[49] Dr Jaya Lakshmi Shreedhar is a health communications expert who specializes in HIV/AIDS and is based in Chennai. Interview on 12 February 2004 in Chennai.

[50] 'Alarming increase in HIV/AIDS cases in Bihar'.

Kolkata School of Tropical Medicine everyday. The report said that the rate of infection among sex workers in Kolkata and its neighbouring areas had gone up from 2 per cent in 1995 to 13 per cent in 1992 and 27.3 per cent in 2001.[51]

In addition to female sex workers and truckers, usually identified as the major carriers, there are also other sections in the country that are rapidly spreading the disease. Aditya Bandopadhyaya, a gay rights' activist, told this author that many gays are HIV-positive, a fact they may not reveal due to social stigma.[52] In addition, there is the New Delhi-based Naz Foundation's finding that nearly four men in 10 recall at least one homosexual encounter.[53] Many would reject the contention that men do have sex with other men and that there is thus a chance of AIDS spreading through the non-traditional path. Acknowledging and thereby taking care of this channel of the spread of AIDS is necessary because reports say that, in Mumbai, an estimated 40 per cent of male sex workers are married.[54] Figure 1.2 shows that people who visit sex-workers do not think they are at risk of contracting HIV/AIDS.

Another channel of HIV/AIDS transmission that many people seem to ignore is through blood and blood products. The World Health Organisation (WHO) estimated in 1998 that perhaps one-fifth of all of India's infections—up to 1 million cases—were due to improperly screened blood and blood products.[55] While normal sexually transmitted diseases (STD) are not as fatal as HIV/AIDS, untreated STDs can increase the risk of HIV transmission as STDs cause mucosal ulceration providing an easy entry for HIV. Approximately 6 to 9 per cent of Indians have some kind of STD,

[51] 'AIDS explosion alert', *The Telegraph*, Calcutta, 2 March 2001.

[52] Interview with Aditya Bandopadhyaya in Hyderabad on 8 February 2004.

[53] Geoffrey Cowley, 'A deadly passage to India', *The Newsweek*, New York, 25 November 2002, available at http://www.blackherbals.com/a_deadly_passage_to_india.htm.

[54] Juliette Terzieff, 'AIDS prevention workers say police harass them as crisis spirals', *San Francisco Chronicle*, San Francisco, 17 November 2002, available at http://www.aegis.com/news/ads/2002/AD022240.html.

[55] Chris Beyrer, 'Accelerating and Disseminating across Asia', *The Washington Quarterly*, Winter 2001, p. 214, available from http://www.twq.com/winter01/beyrer.pdf.

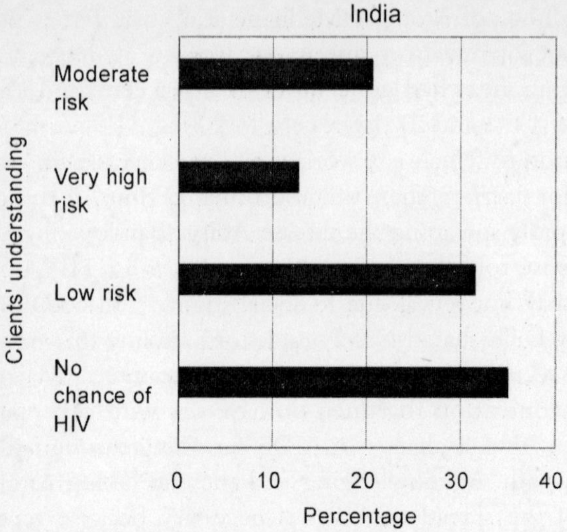

Source: Behavioural Surveillance Survey, 2001.[56]

FIGURE 1.2: DO CLIENTS OF SEX WORKERS BELIEVE THAT THEY ARE RISKING HIV?

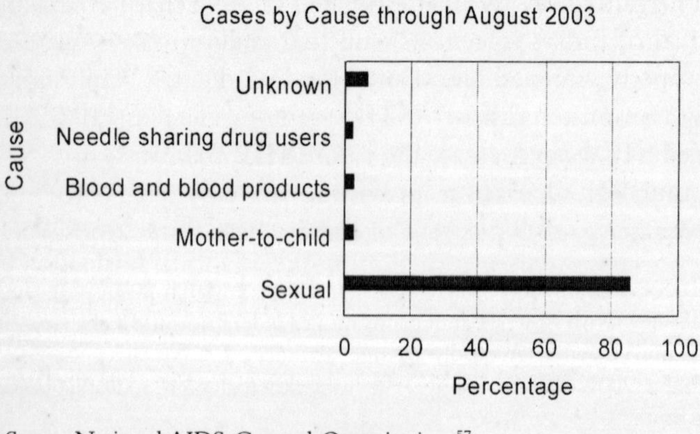

Source: National AIDS Control Organisation.[57]

FIGURE 1.3: HOW DOES HIV SPREAD IN INDIA?

[56] National Baseline General Population Behavioural Surveillance Survey, 2001.

[57] The data is from the National AIDS Control Organisation, India.

with more than 40 million infections every year.[58] This increases their chances of contracting HIV/AIDS. Yet another mode of transmission of HIV/AIDS is from mother to child either through breastfeeding or by birth. See Figure 1.3 to understand how HIV/AIDS spreads in India. The reported rate of mother-to-child infection in India is between 13 and 60 per cent.[59]

It is generally believed that the incidence of drug abuse-related HIV/AIDS is normally found only in the north-eastern parts of India. However, reports suggest that a dispersion of injection drug use has taken place in the major metropolitan cities of Kolkata, Delhi, Chennai, and Mumbai, as well as in other parts of India. While HIV-prevalence is 1 per cent among the IDUs of Kolkata, it is 31 per cent in Chennai.[60] Michael's Care Home in New Delhi, for example, handled 5,200 HIV-positive outpatients and 360 inpatients in 2002–3.[61]

THE FUTURE OF AIDS IN INDIA

The future of AIDS in India could prove to be much worse than is understood by the general public for several reasons, many of which have been explained in the preceding section. These include, high mobility of the population; the nature of the population that is infected which is young and dynamic; rampant poverty in the country which will translate into increased sex work for subsistence and diminished access to health care; and the size of the population which would, at least for some time, complicate attempts at highlighting the issue in the public imagination. What is not a huge concern in the public imagination is unlikely to become a security concern for the political leadership of the country.

The enormous population migration within India and in the region is contributing to the rapid spread of HIV/AIDS. Internal migrants would include:

[58] Suniti Solomon et al., 'HIV in India', p. 20.

[59] Usha Sambamoorthi, Rakkee Thimothy, Wenhui Eei, S Irudaya Rajan, 'Antenatal care and AIDS knowledge among married women', *Economic and Political Weekly*, 14 February 2004, p. 723.

[60] Indrani Gupta et al., 'HIV/AIDS and Development in India', p.14.

[61] Schaffer et al., 'India at the Crossroads', p. 5.

- Permanent and sexual labour migrants within the country
- People dislocated by drought, floods, or other disasters
- People affected by conflict
- Transport workers
- Traders/vendors
- Hotel and tourism workers
- Tourists (e.g. temple tourists)
- Military personnel
- Sex workers
- Trafficked people
- MSM (men who have sex with men)[62]
- Students
- People in transferable jobs

Moreover, with the onset of globalization and the consequent increase in job opportunities in cities, young men and women are thronging to the already overcrowded Indian cities. Many of these migrants from the villages are semi- or fully illiterate, and when they reach a place where they do not have to abide by the strict social norms of the village communities, they often indulge in risky sexual behaviour. Yazdi Italia and I.S. Gilada suggested in 2002 that 29 per cent of the men in Mumbai are single, which further increases the chances of these people visiting sex workers who are plenty in number there.[63] Moreover, in India, the uneven sex ratio can also prove to be a contributing factor in the spread of HIV/AIDS once the disease starts spreading further into the hitherto unaffected parts of the country.[64]

According to a survey by the Mumbai-based International Institute for Population Sciences (IIPS) in 2000–2001 in which it

[62] Ekstrand et al., 'HIV/AIDS in India', p. 53.

[63] Yazdi Italia and I.S. Gilada, ' Invisible Entry of HIV in Rural India, Visibly Distort India's Socioeconomic Fabric', XIV International Conference on AIDS, Barcelona, 7–12 July 2002. Report available at http://www.iaen.org/files.cgi/7035_italia.pdf.

[64] According to the 1991 census of India, of a total of 1,028,610,328 Indians, 532,156,772 were male and only 496,453,556 were female. The sex ratio was 933. Figures available at www.censusindia.net.

examined the prevalence of HIV and the correlates of risk-taking behaviour among migrant workers in two cities, Mumbai and Surat, far fewer migrants had knowledge of sexually transmitted infections (STI) than of HIV/AIDS. The prevalence of risk-taking behaviour (e.g. alcohol consumption, visits to sex workers, and extramarital relationships) was much higher among migrants living alone or with friends as against those living with their own family or with other families.[65] In fact, migration alone is capable of spreading HIV/AIDS into rural India. In a baseline survey of 13 villages in rural Rajasthan, the François-Xavier Bagnoud Center (FXB) found that all men who tested HIV-positive were either migrant workers or had been migrants at some point of time in their life. Three women who were infected were wives of migrant workers.[66]

While truckers cannot strictly be called migrants, they do spend a sufficient amount of time out of their homes to contract the disease. India reportedly has a national highway network of 52,000 km. spanning 35 states. The extended period of time truckers spend away from their families encourages 'high-risk' sexual contacts, thereby increasing the likelihood of their and subsequently their families contracting HIV/AIDS.[67] Dr S.K. Singh of IIPS told this author in an interview that around 80 per cent of the truckers indulge in sexual activities during their journeys. He also said that they were unlikely to carry condoms during journeys.[68]

The fact that 90 per cent of the current infections occur among individuals under the age of 50 means that there are economic implications, but also that the spread of the epidemic among women of childbearing age has significant implications for the further spread of HIV-infections.[69]

Widespread poverty is another crucial factor that will un-

[65] Kamla Gupta and S.K. Singh, 'Social Networking, Knowledge of HIV/AIDS and Risk-Taking Behaviour among Migrant Workers', p. 8, available at http://www.iussp.org/Bangkok2002/S06Gupta.pdf.

[66] Ekstrand et al., 'HIV/AIDS in India', p. 54.

[67] ibid, p. 56.

[68] Interview with S.K. Singh, Reader, IIPS in Mumbai on 4 February 2004.

[69] Sambamoorthi et al., 'Antenatal care and AIDS knowledge among married women', p. 721.

doubtedly increase the spread of HIV/AIDS infection in the country. The number of poor people in India exceeds that of all the states of sub-Saharan Africa combined. Officially, around 25 per cent of Indians live below the poverty line as per the standards set by the National Sample Survey Organisation of the Government of India. Poverty will force some poor women to take up sex work, as many already have, especially in the major metropolitan centres. This will also mean that many of the infected people will not be able to cater to their health needs, eventually succumbing either to related sickness or to HIV/AIDS. Many HIV/AIDS patients will not be able to go to hospitals because, they are poor and also due to an acute lack of public health care facilities. In 1990, India's public health spending was 0.9 per cent of GDP, a figure that did not change during the rest of the decade. The huge difference between public and private health care in India is revealing: in 2000, public expenditure on health accounted for only 18.4 per cent of all health spending.[70]

According to the National Family Health Survey–2, of the married women aged between 15 and 49, living in villages, 53 per cent live in a village with no health facility, and 14 per cent of rural women have to travel at least 5 km. to reach the nearest health facility.[71] This is where the root of the future of the AIDS epidemic is going to be because, given the fact that HIV/AIDS is rapidly spreading to villages, women with no awareness and health facilities will only help in increasing the pace of the spread. A World Bank report published in September 1999 entitled 'India's National AIDS Control Program' shows precisely this danger when it says that India's HIV/AIDS-infection is highly concentrated among the poor and marginalized.[72]

Moreover, the rate of increase of HIV/AIDS in India is extremely high. The rate could be as large as 1–2 million per year

[70] Ekstrand et al., 'HIV/AIDS in India', p. 65.

[71] National Family Health Survey (NFHS-2), 1998–99: India, available at www.nfhsindia.org/data/india/indintro.pdf.

[72] Deepal Jayasekera, 'AIDS becomes a serious health problem in India', 4 May 2001, available at http://www.wsws.org/articles/2001/may2001/aids-m04.shtml.

already, with the total number of infected doubling every 2–3 years. This would mean that if this rate was to continue for the next 6–7 years, there would be as many as 100 million infections by 2010. This stark situation will be compounded by the fact that due to poor health facilities, the mean life after infection is likely to be only 4–5 years.[73] This will easily amount to losing business-persons, servicemen, farmers, truck drivers among others, the real drivers of India's economy, at a mean age of 35. Also, HIV-infected Indians move faster towards AIDS from their HIV sero-positive status to full-blown AIDS compared to HIV/AIDS-infected people anywhere else in the world. The progression of the Indian patient, who does not use antiretroviral therapy (ART), from AIDS to death is twice as fast, at 18 months, whereas it is 33 months in the US.[74] Table 1.6 shows how India's population will be affected by HIV/AIDS in 2000, 2015 and 2050.

TABLE 1.6: POPULATION IN INDIA, ESTIMATED AND PROJECTED WITH AIDS AND WITHOUT AIDS, 2000, 2015 AND 2050

Population (thousands)	2000	2015	2050
With AIDS	1,016,938	1,246,351	1,531,438
Without AIDS	1,020,194	1,264,267	1,612,593

Source: World Population Prospects: The 2002 Revision.[75]

Fifteen years ago, nobody thought that South Africa's HIV/AIDS situation would be what it is today. Similarly, not many people today think that India will soon be in South Africa's position. However, there is some validity in a comparison as 'the principal activities that foster the spread of HIV include polygamous sexual relation in South African society, prostitution along major

[73] Dr Rajan Gupta, 'HIV/AIDS poses a threat to India: A global perspective', available from http://t8web.lanl.gov/people/rajan/AIDS-india/MYWORK/issues.9.99.html.

[74] 'AIDS Spells faster death in India than in US, says study', *Indian Express* (New Delhi), 27 December 2001.

[75] World Population Prospects: The 2002 Revision, available at www.un.org/esa/population/publications/wpp2002/wpp2002annextables.pdf.

transportation arteries, a societal aversion to the use of condoms, and some intravenous drug use in major urban centres.'[76] The problems India faces today are no different.

All indications and examples from other parts of the world do suggest that it is high time India took proactive steps to arrest the further spread of the deadly disease. In fact, much of the damage has already been done and the consequent adverse security repercussions will be felt in the days to come. Thailand's aggressive programme to arrest the disease is probably the best AIDS-prevention programme in the world. Still, one may want to keep in mind that when Thailand started its anti-HIV campaign, adult prevalence was much less there than it is in India today. But even after the successful policies of the Thai government went into effect, statistics suggest that the number of infections continued to rise as the anti-AIDS policies took time to take root.

CONCLUSION

This chapter has broadly made the following arguments:

- Even a mild HIV/AIDS epidemic in the country could have adverse implications for the working-age population of the country;
- While many of the leading think tanks in the world have made studies of how HIV/AIDS can adversely affect a country's security, in India, however, such studies are hard to come by;
- There has been a steady increase in the rate of HIV/AIDS infections in India with two infections in 1986 to 4.5 million in 2002. While official accounts indicate infections close to 5 million, the unofficial accounts indicate figures from 9 to 12 million. A midway point between the two is plausible;
- HIV/AIDS has now changed its 'focus groups' and is increasingly concentrating on the general population and both the rural and the general areas,
- The future of HIV/AIDS in India is extremely worrisome.

[76] Andrew Price-Smith, 'Pretoria's Shadow: The HIV/AIDS pandemic and national security in South Africa', 2002, p. 7, available from http://www.cbaci.org/specialreport4pricesmith.pdf.

CHAPTER 2

HIV/AIDS as a Threat to Security

This chapter will argue that HIV/AIDS is a traditional, human, economic, and societal security threat. The first section will show how the disease is a human security threat, followed by sections on how the disease can also prove to be a threat to India's economic, traditional, and societal security.

HIV/AIDS AS A TRADITIONAL SECURITY THREAT

Traditionally, security has generally been understood as safe borders, military force strength, political stability, ability to project power, etc. This study attempts to show that howsoever one may define security, HIV/AIDS will prove to be a threat. In the first place, it is necessary to see how HIV/AIDS can prove to be a traditional security threat.

This section will attempt to show that HIV/AIDS can eventually affect the military population of India, interfere with the country's global peace-keeping missions, which can be considered to be a subtle way of power projection, lead to law and order problems and political instability, and trouble international migration and cross-border activities like trade.

Given the fact that military training is supposed to instil a sense of discipline among its personnel, it is generally believed that soldiers are less likely to be infected by the HIV virus than the general population. This is not only false but in fact the reverse is true. Soldiers have higher chances of contracting HIV/AIDS than the general public because of the following factors:

- Opportunity for risky behaviour

- Risk-taking ethos and other attitudinal factors
- Separation from their communities
- Duties which force them to be geographically mobile, going far away from home for a long period leading to sex deprivation[1]
- Large concentrations of troops may attract sex workers, especially when deployed in areas of material scarcity
- Alcohol and other drugs used to cope with the pressures of military life further increase the chances of unprotected sexual intercourse
- Sexual activity, consensual or forced, typically increases in times of conflict[2]
- They belong to the right age group to contract HIV/AIDS

A soldier once infected with HIV/AIDS, having lost all hopes of a peaceful retirement, is likely to engage in reckless behaviour and may go on to earn money through other means to pay his medical expenses. Having such soldiers in sensitive and key installations could prove to be dangerous.

India has about 1.3 million military personnel. Since India has a large pool of potential recruits, the disease is unlikely to create a military security problem. However, the lack of recruits is not the only way a nation's military can be threatened by HIV/AIDS. There are many more ways a country's military can derail national security which it is supposed to safeguard. As mentioned earlier, in a country like India, military personnel who are infected by HIV/AIDS and who would not divulge it due to the fear of losing their job and the social stigma attached to it could jeopardize military prowess and preparedness.

There does not yet seem to be any comprehensive data gathering on the extent of the HIV/AIDS infection in the Indian military. When contacted by this author, medical officers of the Indian military in New Delhi said that there was no such comprehensive data, but there were enough medical facilities to look after those

[1] 'AIDS and the military: UNAIDS point of view', May 1998, available at www.worldbank.org/wbi/aidsleadership/ dls_AIDS_military_may14.pdf.

[2] Elbe, 'Strategic implications of HIV/AIDS', p. 20.

who did get infected by HIV/AIDS. An Indian army general acknowledged in a talk show on New Delhi Television (NDTV) that there is a 2 per cent infection rate among military personnel who donate blood.[3] A newspaper report in 1998 claimed that 6,000 members of the Indian army tested HIV-positive.[4] After the Cambodian peacekeeping mission, 45 Indian soldiers had tested HIV-positive.[5] The prevalence of HIV among the Cambodian military ranges between 6 and 17 per cent.[6] Reports have also mentioned that some personnel of India's Border Security Force (BSF) have tested HIV-positive.[7] However, these small figures in no way represent the depth of the HIV problem in the Indian military. On the other hand, there are reports that Pakistan-backed militants are spreading the disease in Jammu & Kashmir which is not a highly infected state. A newspaper report claimed in March 2004 that the increase in HIV/AIDS rates in the state has been traced to foreign tourists from Pakistan and Afghanistan who may have been spreading this deadly virus through homosexual or heterosexual contact.'[8]

Cedric Fernandez who has extensive experience with HIV/AIDS victims in India's north-east argues that many Border Security Force (BSF) personnel deployed in places like Manipur are HIV-positive due to the fact that many female sex workers (FSWs) with no other means of livelihood approach the paramilitary forces offering them cheap sex.[9] Having been away from home for extended periods of time, soldiers do enter into risky sexual contacts, often contracting HIV/AIDS.

[3] It was discussed in a talk show by Rajdeep Sardesai on New Delhi Television at 10.00 p.m. on 12 July 2004. This was conveyed to this author by Kanti Bajpai in a personal communication later.

[4] Elbe, 'Strategic implications of HIV/AIDS', p. 19.

[5] Ibid., p. 41.

[6] Ibid., p. 19.

[7] 'HIV positive soldier challenges dismissal in court', 26 October 2003, Agence France-Presse, accessed at http://www.aegis.com/news/afp/2003/AF031095.html

[8] 'Terrorists spreading AIDS in J&K'. 31 March 2004 *Daily Excelsior* (Jammu), available at http://www.dailyexcelsior.com/web1/04mar31/news.htm

[9] Interview with Cedric Fernandez.

Also, police personnel deployed in India's metropolitan cities stand every chance of contracting HIV/AIDS. *The Times of India* reported in 2003 that 450 police personnel had tested HIV-positive since 1991, 18 of whom had died.[10] Many of the health workers this author talked to in Pune, Mumbai and even Chennai share the view that the number could be much higher given the fact that police personnel in the red-light districts of Mumbai and Pune, as is the case everywhere else, have chances of having free sex with sex workers, and most of these policemen are unlikely to carry condoms while on duty. Ms. Namrata Chauhan says that she has witnessed a number of policemen visiting brothels. She claims it is very regular among them.[11] UNAIDS findings suggest that in peacetime, STD infection rates among the armed forces are generally 2–5 times higher than in comparable civilian populations, and the difference could be even greater in times of conflict.[12] Given the fact that those with STDs can contract HIV faster, the Indian military is fast proceeding toward greater rates of HIV/AIDS-infections.

Soon there will be in place a regional HIV/AIDS cooperation programme between the Indian military and the Pacific Command's Center of Excellence at the US Surgeon's Office.[13] This certainly means that Indian military planners are taking cognizance of the problem of HIV/AIDS infection within the armed forces. What, however, remains to be seen is whether the Indian military can think differently from their counterparts in the civilian administration who are still to fully comprehend the implications of the dangerous situation in the country.

One thing that the HIV/AIDS prevalence rate in the African militaries has made abundantly clear is that peacekeeping missions can both spread and contract HIV/AIDS. Peacekeepers have very

[10] 'Mumbai police face mandatory HIV testing', 28 January 2004, available at www.worldvision.org/worldvision/pr.nsf/ stable/update_india_012804.

[11] Personal email communication from Namrata Chauhan.

[12] 'AIDS and the military: UNAIDS point of view', May 1998, available at http://www.worldbank.org/wbi/aidsleadership/dls_AIDS_military_may14.pdf.

[13] Josy Joseph, 'Indo–US defense cooperation on HIV/AIDS program', 11 March 2004, Rediff Special.

often acted as vectors of HIV/AIDS, spreading the virus among the population in areas of deployment. While the risk of the forces contracting HIV/AIDS during deployment may reduce a contributing state's willingness to participate in peacekeeping operations, states may also become less willing to host peacekeeping operations.[14] They may also refuse to send their peacekeepers to serve alongside troops from countries which have a high prevalence of HIV/AIDS.

In 1995, the US State Department observed that, 'world wide peacekeeping operations may pose a danger of spreading HIV... peacekeepers could both be a source of HIV-infection to local populations and be infected by them, thus becoming a source of the infection when they return home.'[15] The French also reportedly found that a tour of duty abroad increased the risk of contracting HIV by a factor of five.[16] It has been observed that in Sierra Leone and Liberia, peacekeepers have been among the main agents for spreading HIV. A US intelligence analyst warned that US military forces deployed in support of humanitarian and peacekeeping operations in developing countries could be at risk from infectious diseases, including HIV.[17]

HIV/AIDS can give rise to serious problems in bilateral relations and defence agreements. For example, as the Philippine government's defence agreement with the US was about to end in 1991, activists accused the US forces of introducing and spreading HIV/AIDS in the country.[18] India has a commendable track record of sending troops on international peacekeeping missions. It is therefore not out of place to say that India may also one day face similar accusations.

The length of duty, without rotation, in an acutely HIV/AIDS-infected country, can also lead peacekeepers to contract the disease. It was reported that some Nigerian peacekeepers who were on duty without rotation for up to 3 years in Sierra Leone had

[14] Elbe, 'Strategic implications of HIV/AIDS', p. 39.

[15] 'HIV/AIDS as a Security Issue', ICG Report, p. 22.

[16] Ibid.

[17] Ibid.

[18] Elbe, 'Strategic implications of HIV/AIDS', p. 26.

contracted the disease, the rate of which was later correlated with the length of duty increasing from 7 per cent after one year to 10 per cent after two years to 15 per cent after three years.[19] On the other hand, countries which never had a reported case of HIV/AIDS have subsequently seen dramatic increases in the instance of the disease after a UN-led peacekeeping operation in those countries. For example, East Timor never had a reported case of HIV/AIDS till a UN force arrived there. Similarly, in Cambodia, the prevalence of HIV/AIDS increased following the arrival of the UN transitional authority.[20] Such instances have forced the UN to buy condoms for its peacekeepers, as it did in Sierra Leone and East Timor. Some host countries have gone even further. In 2001, the government of Eritrea demanded that peacekeepers deployed in the country should be screened for HIV/AIDS.[21]

However, in an age where the UN's authority is rapidly decreasing, it is not easy to enforce such screening rules given the paucity of available troops and the potential non-compliance of many contributing states, though the UNSC resolution 1308 urges countries to screen the soldiers for HIV/AIDS.[22]

Will HIV/AIDS affect political stability? It is likely to, in the longer run. The social and economic impact of infectious diseases is likely to intensify the struggle for political power and for scarce state resources, especially in a country like India where fighting among the people for essential commodities like water takes place on a daily basis. [23]

In an international trading system where the competition for markets in the various countries and disputes over accepting and rejecting goods on the flimsiest of grounds have become the order

[19] Ibid., p. 41.

[20] Ibid., p. 40.

[21] Ibid., p. 43.

[22] United Nations Security Council Resolution 1308 (2000), adopted by the Security Council at its 4172nd meeting, on 17 July 2000, available at http://www.casy.org/engdocs/UNseccounl_00.htm.

[23] John C. Gannon, Chairman, NIC, 'The Global Infectious Diseases Threat and its Implications for the United States', available at http://www.cia.gov/cia/reports/nie/report/nie99-17d.html.

of the day, infectious disease-related embargoes and restrictions on travel and immigration will cause friction among and between developed and developing countries.[24]

HIV/AIDS could also create problems between neighbouring countries. For example, according to a Red Cross study, at least 10 per cent of Nepalese workers from the far western region, who arrive in India searching for employment contract HIV/AIDS after having unsafe sex in India.[25] Usha Koirala, Nepal's leading AIDS activist, says that at least 60 per cent of HIV-positive people in the country had returned from India where they had had unsafe sex.[26] Nepal has not made a bilateral issue out of its AIDS problem as it cannot afford to do so. But there is a lot of talk about India exporting HIV/AIDS to Nepal. This can only increase the already strong anti-Indian feeling in Nepal.

HIV/AIDS AS A HUMAN SECURITY THREAT

Kanti Bajpai defines human security as protection from direct and indirect threats to the personal safety and well-being of the individual.[27] Going by that definition, HIV/AIDS *prima facie* constitutes a human security threat because the HIV/AIDS-related suffering and consequent untimely death constitutes undeniable suffering and loss of dignity for a person.

HIV/AIDS thus destroys human security, both at the individual and at the collective level, by way of causing individual suffering and death, causing the HIV/AIDS victims to contract other opportunistic diseases, and fall prey to the normal Indian practice of making them social outcasts. It kills people at an extremely productive and reproductive age and creates demographic problems within the country (see Table 2.1).

[24] Ibid.

[25] Sudeeshna Sarkar, 'Nepalese workers contracting HIV in India: Report', *Hindustan Times Online,* 19 August 2003.

[26] 'Alarm over AIDS on India-Nepal border', *Agence France* Press, 23 August 2000, available at http://w3.whosea.org/healthnews/ie24aug.htm

[27] Kanti Bajpai, 'Human Security: Concept and Measurement', Kroc Institute Occasional Paper, August 2000, available at http://www.nd.edu/~krocinst/ocpapers/op_19_1.PDF.

TABLE 2.1: EXCESS NUMBER OF DEATHS ESTIMATED AND PROJECTED WITH AIDS *Vs.* WITHOUT AIDS IN INDIA BY THE HIV/AIDS EPIDEMIC, 1980–2000, 2000–15 AND 2015–50

	1980–2000		2000–15		2015–50	
India	Excess deaths (thousands)	Percentage increase	Excess deaths (thousands)	Percentage increase	Excess deaths (thousands)	Percentage increase
	2,665	1	12,358	10	49,504	12

Source: World Population Prospects: The 2002 Revision.[28]

What is assumed here at a very fundamental and conceptual level, as Andrew Price-Smith says, is that any agent that directly threatens to destroy a significant proportion of a state's population is a direct threat to that state's security.[29] It may not destroy a significant proportion of India's population in the near future, not because the number of people infected by HIV/AIDS is low, but because the country's population is huge. That certainly is no consolation because as the argument stands, it does contribute to the suffering of large numbers of Indians, thus making it a human security threat of national proportions.

At an individual level, falling prey to HIV/AIDS would mean being stigmatized by the community that one lives in (a detailed discussion on HIV/AIDS-related stigma is taken up at a later stage) because, for most people in India, sex is a taboo subject and since most HIV-infections in India result from sexual activity, HIV/AIDS is also a taboo subject. Thus, a person who is infected by HIV/AIDS will be deemed a social outcast and not allowed to participate in public life. Freedom of movement is often highly restricted, and human dignity is non-existent. Mostly for no fault of theirs, women who fall victim to HIV/AIDS—having contracted it from their husbands—as a number of surveys have shown, are

[28] 'World Population Prospects: The 2002 Revision', p. 85, available at www.un.org/esa/population/publications/wpp2002/wpp2002annextables.PDF.

[29] Price-Smith, 'Pretoria's Shadow', p. 3.

victimized more than their husbands who gave them the disease in the first place. Moreover, if they lose their husbands first, it would most probably mean loss of economic status. They are likely to migrate to cities looking for jobs and will most probably end up in the sex industry.

The human security of an HIV/AIDS-infected person is further jeopardized when he/she is not able to get adequate medical care. An increase in the number of HIV/AIDS cases in the days to come will mean that hospitals will (many of them already do) discriminate against these infected with HIV/AIDS. Dr C. Gilks in his paper 'Impact on health system in India' says that HIV/AIDS patients will ultimately have a major impact on the health care system as a whole as HIV/AIDS patients take up 25 per cent of all hospital beds, 60 per cent of all physician time, and 44 per cent of all healthcare expenditure.[30] What this means is that patients with other sicknesses will not receive adequate care as there is already an acute lack of health infrastructure in the country. Moreover, HIV/AIDS also attacks and destroys the human immune system and consequently allows many other opportunistic diseases like TB to take root in the human body.

Nicholas Eberstadt makes two observations in his article in *Foreign Affairs*. First, even if countries had funds, they would probably not spend them on HIV/AIDS because the huge costs involved in distributing the treatment (even assuming that the drugs were given away free) would often be more than the economic value to governments of the lives thus saved. Second, until some kind of cure is discovered, most people with HIV/AIDS in the developing world are not going to be saved.[31] This analysis throws up many disturbing questions. How far is such an analysis true for a huge and poor country like India which has an equally poor track record of the health care of its people? Till the time there is an influential section in the society committed to virtues like human dignity

[30] Dr C. Gilks, 'Impact on the Health system in India', Summaries of Publications from UNDP Asia-Pacific Regional Project on HIV and Development, available at http://www.hivundp.apdip.net/Regional/Publication%20The%20Economics%20of%20AIDS.pdf.

[31] Eberstadt, 'The Future of AIDS', p. 44.

and human rights, will the government take responsibility for the HIV/AIDS-infected? Eberstadt's second conclusion is even more pessimistic, which essentially means that in a country like India, HIV/AIDS will definitely prove to be life-threatening. Whether one takes the sheer numbers of people affected, or the living conditions of the infected people, or the lack of human dignity they get in society, HIV/AIDS is a human security threat.

HIV/AIDS AS AN ECONOMIC SECURITY THREAT

While there is no comprehensive study that has mapped the economic costs and losses of HIV/AIDS across the length and breadth of India, it is sufficiently clear by now to those looking closely at the issue that HIV/AIDS will have both long-term and short-term adverse implications on the Indian economy. This section looks at how HIV/AIDS will adversely affect India's Gross Domestic Product (GDP), labour and industrial productivity, household economy, foreign direct investment, how the transport system and migration spread the disease and how they in turn are affected by it. At the end of the section, the results of some surveys already done will be presented.

We do know that HIV/AIDS will definitely have adverse impacts on the Indian economy as has been demonstrated by the various studies already done in many parts of India. Calculating the economic costs of HIV/AIDS would require calculating how much less a population would earn due to HIV, how much more it would be obliged to devote to covering the needs of AIDS victims, and the present value of the differences in these amounts. Eberstradt concludes that there just isn't the data needed for such a study.[32]

Indrani Gupta writes that a number of studies have come to the conclusion that the costs of HIV/AIDS on the Indian economy calculated mainly in terms of medical costs (due to treatment of secondary infections) and loss of productivity would amount to as much as 1 per cent of GDP.[33] However, such studies have not

[32] Ibid, p. 39.

[33] Indrani Gupta, 'Do we still need more evidence?' *Seminar,* 520, December 2002, p. 24.

included many essential factors like the cost of drugs and retaining workers.[34] A study by David Bloom et al., indicated a total cost burden on the country of around $ 11 billion by 2000.[35] Eberstadt suggests that, in India, Gross National Product without

> HIV would be almost 170 per cent higher in 2025 than in 2000—with growth driven both by a larger workforce and by increasing worker productivity. Under the mild epidemic scenario, GNP would still rise substantially—but by about a third less over that quarter-century than the 'no-aids' baseline would be predicted. If there was an intermediate epidemic, predicted GNP in 2025 would be 40 per cent lower than the baseline scenario; national output would still grow, but growth would be cut by three-fourths over the next 25 years.[36]

A World Bank study suggests that even an adult prevalence rate of 10 per cent may reduce the growth of national income up to a third.[37] WHO estimates that if the infection rates are above 20 per cent, a nation's GDP may decline by 1 per cent per year.[38]

India's life expectancy is projected to increase to 66.3 per cent during 2010–15, to 67.8 per cent during 2020–25 and to 73.8 per cent during 2045–50. However, it is also projected by the UN that AIDS will reduce life expectancy by 2–4 per cent by 2050. Thus the nation will stand to lose its biggest assets—the working-age population. This is probably the clearest example of how economic security can be a threat to the country's national security.

The World Bank said in 1997 that if India maintained its current level of health care subsidies, a severe AIDS epidemic would increase government expenditure by about $2 billion per year by 2010. If there is a hike in the subsidies to the 50 per cent level, an epidemic of the same proportions would increase annual government health expenditure by an additional $30 billion.[39] This is despite the fact that, as a study of 2000 points out, India's public health expenditure

[34] Gorden, 'The Next Wave of HIV/AIDS', p. 20.

[35] Indrani Gupta, 'Do we still need more evidence?' p. 24.

[36] Eberstadt, 'The Future of AIDS', p. 41.

[37] 'HIV/AIDS as a Security Issue', ICG report, p. 4.

[38] Mark Schneider and Michael Moodie, 'The Destabilastion impacts of HIV/AIDS', May 2002, available at www.csis.org.

[39] Cited in Indrani Gupta et al., p. 13.

is no more than 1.2 per cent of its GDP, placing it among the lowest quintile countries.[40] Government expenditure on health is no more than 20 per cent of the total health expenditure in the country.

According to UNDP estimates, income losses due to the death of skilled adults will cost the country Rs 3,52,000 per case, and medical care and income losses could work out to be $352 billion by 2000, which amounts to a full 5 per cent of India's GDP.[41]

Anand, Pandav and Nath, who have done remarkable studies on the economic costs of HIV/AIDS in India, calculated that considering that the total cumulative number of HIV-infected persons in India until 1995 was 1.5 million (low estimate), 2.5 million (medium estimate), 4.5 million (high estimate), the estimated total annual cost (in billion rupees) under the low, medium, and high assumptions was 6.73, 20.16 and 59.19, respectively. The components of the cost of HIV/AIDS in their study were cost of treatment and loss in productivity. They do admit that all costs of HIV/AIDS were not taken into consideration.[42]

Indrani Gupta et al., studied the health and treatment costs for 1999 and calculated that Rs 2,045 crores would have been spent in 1999 in India. Moreover, 'this was the minimum expenditures or costs that would have taken place in one year if only 2.8 per cent of the individuals are on antiretroviral treatment and only half of the new infection[s] in 1999 display any opportunistic infection.'[43] A report by Maria Ekstrand et al., in 2003 titled 'HIV/AIDS in India' says:

> during the late 1990s, estimates of the total annual cost of HIV/AIDS in India ranged from 7 billion to 60 billion rupees. These figures were obtained by calculating the average cost per AIDS case (cost of opportunistic infections (OI) treatment and lost productivity) and multiplying the estimates of the total cumulative number of HIV-infected

[40] Deepal Jayasekara, 'AIDS becomes a serious health problem in India'.

[41] Mitu Varma, 'India—Health: AIDS Watch, Poverty Watch', 26 September 1997, available at http://www.aegis.com/news/ips/1997/IP970908.html.

[42] K. Anand, C.S. Pandav and L.M. Nath, 'Impact of HIV/AIDS on the National Economy of India', *Health Policy*, vol. 49, no. 3, June 1999, pp. 195–205.

[43] Indrani Gupta et al., p. 13.

persons. The researchers concluded that AIDS costs India roughly 1 per cent of GDP per year because of lost productivity and treatment of OIs. However, the study did not include numerous factors such as the cost of antiretroviral therapy (ART), strengthening the health care system, and the retraining of workers. Although studies often use prevalence and economic structures to assess the impact of HIV/AIDS on economic growth, this approach does not always yield precise estimates.[44]

What many people forget when calculating GDP loss due to HIV/AIDS is the labour of the women workforce. Franklyn Lisk rightly points out: 'women bear and care for the workforce, present and future, as well as taking part in it themselves. The fact that much of women's work may not be counted in GDP does not alter society's economic dependence on them. It follows, therefore, that if women are vulnerable so are those who depend on them, from the household to the national economy.'[45] Another sector on which exact data is not available is the informal sector. Vague though the exact nature of its economic contribution is, it is this sector that is likely to suffer the most due to HIV/AIDS because of poor health facilities, lack of social protection, and greater job and financial insecurity.[46]

Ajay Mahal and David Bloom examined the annual treatment costs of HIV/AIDS in nine Asian countries in the mid-1990s and came to the conclusion that these costs were more than twice the per capita income in each country. In India, they say, the ratio of treatment costs to per capita income was 2.2. Their estimates did not, however, include the costs of ARVs.[47] A World Bank estimate says that the money used to treat one AIDS patient with the protease inhibitor cocktail would keep 400 children in school for a year.[48]

[44] Ekstrand et al., 'HIV/AIDS in India'.

[45] Franklyn Lisk, 'Labour Market and Employment Implications of HIV/AIDS', June 2002, ILO Programme on HIV/AIDS and the World of Work, Geneva, June 2002, p. 9.

[46] Ibid., p. 3.

[47] Ajay Mahal, 'Economic implications of inertia on HIV/AIDS and Benefits of Action', *Economic and Political Weekly*, 6 March 2004, p. 1051.

[48] 'HIV/AIDS as a Security Issue', ICG report, p. 18.

HIV/AIDS will almost certainly affect the monetary savings of a nation. An increase in the consumption of medicine as a result of HIV/AIDS will see a decrease in domestic savings, which will then indicate a fall in capital formation leading to a potentially large adverse effect on per capita income over the long term.[49] Savings rates could also decline if people expect to live a fewer number of years due to HIV/AIDS, because they feel less need to save to meet their old-age consumption needs.[50]

Malcolm McPherson, Deborah Hoover, and Donald Snodgrass write:

> Individuals who are HIV-positive increase their consumption, in part to combat the effects of disease, and in part, because the prospect of premature death raises the opportunity cost of time. These changes lower the supply of investible resources, at both the individual and national levels, and reduce the efficiency with which the existing stock of productive assets is used. Those effects, in turn, lower the rate of growth of per capita incomes, setting off a further cycle of declining savings and investment.[51]

Ajay Mahal claims that:

> high rates of AIDS related deaths among more educated age groups could directly act to reduce the stock of human capital, as well as indirectly, because people will have less of an incentive to acquire costly educational capital, if they do not expect to live long enough to enjoy substantial gains from acquiring it. The future of educational capital could also be affected if children whose parents die prematurely due to AIDS face economic bottlenecks in efforts to continue their education.[52]

[49] Thiyam Bharat, 'HIV/AIDS and Socio-Economy', 8 July 2002, available at http://www.manipuronline.com/Features/July2002/hivandsocioeconomy 08_1.htm.

[50] Ajay Mahal, 'Economic implications of inertia on HIV/AIDS and Benefits of Action', p. 1050.

[51] Malcolm McPherson, Deborah Hoover, and Donald Snodgrass, 'The Impact on Economic Growth in Africa of Rising Costs and Labor Productivity Losses Associated with HIV/AIDS', Working Paper, Kennedy School of Government, Harvard University, 2000, available at http://www.cid.harvard.edu/caer2/htm/content/papers/bns/dp79bn.htm, pp. 11–12.

[52] Mahal, 'Economic implications of inertia on HIV/AIDS and Benefits of Action', p. 1050.

Given that there are not enough health care facilities to look after HIV/AIDS victims in the country due to the ever-increasing rush in the number of HIV/AIDS patients going to hospitals for treatment, individuals seeking health care for other diseases can be left without care. There is already evidence of this from states like Tamil Nadu and Manipur.[53]

One fact that everyone holds as true is that HIV/AIDS will negatively influence sectors that are labour-intensive, medicare fields such as health care and health insurance, and sectors that may be particularly sensitive to the risk of ill health (such as tourism).[54]

The seriousness of this threat to a nation's economic security is further compounded by the fact that the mean age of the people currently coming to hospitals is between 25 and 30 years.[55] Moreover, the population that is the most sexually active and by implication most likely to get infected by HIV/AIDS is also India's most economically productive. Thus HIV/AIDS will not only reduce India's per capita productivity and labour supply, it will also result in the loss of primary bread-winners in families, leading to further problems in the victims' families.[56] It is a double-edged sword in the sense that, on the one hand, the working-age population will stop working and, on the other, the non-working-age population will have to pay for their medical expenses.

Malcolm McPherson, Senior Fellow in Development at Harvard University, considers the following to be some of the areas where the macroeconomic impacts of HIV/AIDS will be felt:

- Individuals/farm households (shorter horizons, increased uncertainty about future, higher current costs → reduce investment)
- Business (higher short-term costs such as health, training,

[53] Indrani Gupta et al., p. 13.

[54] Mahal, 'Economic implications of inertia on HIV/AIDS and Benefits of Action', p. 1050.

[55] Dr. Rajan Gupta, 'HIV/AIDS poses a threat to India'.

[56] 'The HIV/AIDS Crisis in India', *South Asia Monitor*, CSIS, available at www.csis.org/saprog/sam58.pdf.

disrupted work schedules and prospects of falling future demand → reduce investment)

- Government (higher recurrent costs such as health, education, redundancy payments and prospects of declining future revenue → reduce investment)

And because of the disease a country would:

- Lose advantages of specialization
- Lose complementarities created by skill agglomeration
- Lose competitiveness as scale shrinks and unit costs rise
- Give an opportunity to investors to exercise the option of waiting (or leaving)[57]

In a survey conducted in 2000 and 2001 in Tamil Nadu by Dorisamy Palanigounder et al., it was found among other things that:

- Median direct costs of treatment and services in a reference period of six months is Rs 6000;
- Medical cost comprises 70 per cent of direct cost;
- Direct cost significantly increases with stages of illness and household income;
- The average financial burden of treatment, measured as the percentage of household income spent on treatment and services, is 49 per cent;
- The burden is high in low-income households;
- The number of clients reporting loss of income was 46 per cent at the beginning of the survey; and
- HIV/AIDS leads to depletion of savings and productive assets and increases household indebtedness.

Costs in this study were calculated as direct costs and indirect costs with the former comprising doctors' fees, hospital charges, medicine and tests, travel, food, lodging, and rituals, and the latter

[57] Malcolm McPherson, 'The Macroeconomic Impact of HIV/AIDS', 29 January 2003, available at www.iris.umd.edu/ppc_IDEAS/HIV_AIDS/01_29_03.asp.

consisting of loss of income and fringe benefits, and workdays lost and change of job.[58]

SETBACKS IN THE GLOBAL MARKET PLACE?

To say that HIV/AIDS will prove to be a setback for India in the globalized marketplace may seem far-fetched but while it is true that the adverse impacts of HIV/AIDS are yet to be seen as a threat to FDI flow into India or to the country's foreign trade, what can be said is that in a highly competitive international trading system that is rapidly emerging in the global arena, diseases like HIV/AIDS can and will deter investments, investors and business opportunities. Investors may wait when they come to know that the spread of HIV/AIDS is likely to adversely affect the cost structure of any investment they are contemplating. This is also true of the domestic investors because 'as the perceived costs of dealing with the spread of HIV/AIDS rise, the rates of investment tend to decline.... Thus while the spread of HIV/AIDS induces the need for higher rates of investment to help maintain worker productivity, it erodes the means by which such investment can be financed.'[59]

In an age where mere rumours can induce capital flight overnight, investment capital might easily move to regions with lower morbidity and mortality rates, leading to declines in economic growth and the subsequent inability of countries to sustain their place in the competitive international market.[60] The situation is even more precarious for a Third World country like India. Given the sheer size of the population, India and China may continue to fill the gap of labour supply in so far as the disease remains among the rural and lower-skilled people. However, as the disease spreads to the young, educated, urban professionals, the higher will be the

[58] Duraisamy Palanigounder, 'Economic impact of HIV/AIDS on patients and households in South India: costs and burden on households and coping strategies', available at www.iaen.org/ files.cgi/9838_EcoImpact-HIV-AIDS-SouthIndia.doc.

[59] Price-Smith, 'Pretoria's Shadow', p. 16.

[60] Elbe, 'Strategic implications of HIV/AIDS', p. 149.

economic costs.[61] Dr. Ashok Rao of the Freedom Foundation, who this author spoke with in Bangalore, suggests that the IT industry in Bangalore could be one such area of concern. For many of the youngsters working in the IT city, with higher disposable incomes, lack of family control, unmarried status, and increased prosperity may mean the freedom to indulge in casual sex and thus to contract HIV/AIDS, putting at risk both the IT industry in Bangalore and the international business the city gets.[62]

Specialized areas such as IT, nursing, and tourism could be hard hit. Widespread prevalence of HIV/AIDS in a city or a country can also adversely affect international decisions about direct investment, technology transfer and, more importantly, personnel allocation.[63] Ashok Rao says that many of the patients are Information Technology (IT) professionals and servicemen. He has discussed the implementation of prevention strategies with IT firms in Bangalore. Many call girls, he says, are poor village girls who cater to metropolitan high-class workers. Their awareness and education levels are unlikely to be high. Because city professionals also practise, sex within a closed group, it is possible for one of them to contact the infection from a sex worker and pass it on to all others in the group later.[64]

While international migration can bring HIV/AIDS to the country, as in the case of Kerala, HIV/AIDS may also adversely affect international migration.[65] More than 1 lakh Indians leave each year to work in other countries, 80 per cent of whom are unskilled. There were around 1.5 million Indian migrant workers in West Asia in 1991; by 1995 there were over 4 million. 'The Gulf is home to some 3.6 million Indians, of whom the largest number, 1.5 million, live in Saudi Arabia. There are 1 million in the United Arab Emirates, almost half a million each in Kuwait

[61] Gorden, 'The Next Wave of HIV/AIDS', p. 4.

[62] Interview with Ashok Rao in Bangalore on 12 February 2004.

[63] Ibid.

[64] Ibid.

[65] India HIV/AIDS Alliance and Kerala State Management Agency state that 80 per cent of reported AIDS cases are 'migration related'. See for details Ekstrand et al., 'HIV/AIDS in India', p. 54.

and Oman, and around 1 lakh each in Bahrain and Qatar.'[66] It is highly likely that in the event of an HIV/AIDS epidemic in India, the Gulf countries may put a ban on Indian workers, especially from the worst-hit states, as labour is easily available from other low HIV-prevalent countries such as Pakistan and Bangladesh.

HIV/AIDS can also cause a country to lose its competitive edge in an indirect manner. The rampant spread of the disease could limit a country's spending on higher education, subsequently draining its population of technical skills. If India loses such technical skills in competitive sectors like IT, the outcome could be disastrous.

India's industrial hubs and special economic zones are also not safe from the adverse impacts of HIV/AIDS due primarily to the fact that a large part of the spread of HIV/AIDS today is in the industrial and agricultural workforce which is reportedly 200-million strong in India. Most of the industrial hubs and economic zones are surrounded by shanty towns and slums. People living in these hubs often resort to cheap sex with Commercial Sex Workers (CSW)[67] and so pose a threat not only to industrial productivity but they also carry the infection back to their villages. Dr S.K. Singh of IIPS, who has extensive experience in assessing the impact of HIV on industry, says that when the Enron power plant was functional in Maharashtra, there were a large number of sex workers in the neighbouring areas who had come specially to cater to the sexual needs of the workers there. [68] Such practices are likely to be the rule rather than the exception.

Orissa's Ganjam district not only has a very high rate of HIV/AIDS among the locals, but it also has about 1 lakh persons from the district engaged in menial jobs in various factories and construction sites in Gujarat and Maharashtra.[69] According to official figures, Vadodara in Gujarat, one of India's premier industrial cities,

[66] George Iype, 'No longer Mecca for Prosperity', 7 July 2004, available at http://specials.rediff.com/news/2004/jul/07spec2.htm

[67] Dr Rajan Gupta, 'HIV/AIDS poses a threat to India'.

[68] Interview with Dr. S K Singh.

[69] Sisir Panigrahy, 'AIDS spurt in Orissa district raises alarm', *Indian Express*, New Delhi, 15 January 2002.

has more than 6,000 HIV/AIDS-infections.[70] Unofficial figures could be higher, and the migrant population that works there may have carried the virus back to other states and non-AIDS regions. Moreover, 'Gujarat, being an industrially-developed state, is highly vulnerable to AIDS owing to its floating population, mostly comprising [*sic*] migrant labourers', doctors in Gujarat confirm.[71]

Surat, yet another industrial town of India, famous for diamonds and infamous for the plague that the city experienced in 1994, has a large number of HIV/AIDS victims, and the threat is growing. A survey in the city revealed that as many as 5,000 migrant labourers who work in Surat are infected with the deadly virus. Some voluntary organizations believe that the figure may be 10 times higher than what we may come across in random screenings. It is reported that migrant labourers there are particularly vulnerable because they fall in the sexually active age group of 16 to 35. Since only 15 per cent of them have their families with them,[72] there is every chance of their contracting HIV/AIDS and passing it on to their families back home, in the process jeopardizing the industrial activity in the city, if not now, then some time later.

Raipur, the capital of the state of Chhattisgarh, has a number of large cement factories. Reportedly, more than a thousand trucks stop in the city each day. Truckers, industry and migrant labour seem to have driven the city towards a high prevalence of HIV/AIDS. Almost 30 per cent of the local doctors have come across an HIV-positive case. Doctors at the Raipur medical college speak of getting one new HIV-infected case each day and almost 40 persons on regular follow-ups.[73]

The problem is compounded by a lack of awareness among the victims about HIV/AIDS. The Mumbai-based International

[70] Prathima Nandakumar, 'Vadodara has 6,000 HIV positive cases', *Times of India*, New Delhi, 17 May 2003.

[71] Ibid.

[72] Mohurya Chaudhuri, 'Indian Migrant Workers: Sweatshop Conditions/ Ignorance Lead to AIDS Epidemic', 22 February 2002, available at http://www.comminit.com/strategicthinking/commentary/sld-2136.html.

[73] Mail from Dr A.K. Agarwal, Shram Shakti Project, Raipur, Madhya Pradesh to the Yahoo AIDS India Forum in 2002.

Institute for Population Sciences examined HIV prevalence and the correlates of risk-taking behaviour among migrant workers in Surat and Mumbai. In a 2000–1 survey, it found that not many migrants had adequate knowledge of HIV/AIDS though the number of people who were aware of it was far greater than those who were aware of STIs. The survey also found that the prevalence of risk-taking behaviour was higher among migrants living alone or with friends versus these living with their own family or with other families.[74]

Another category whose losses are unlikely to figure comprehensively in India's GDP losses is the household sector. The inevitable impacts of HIV/AIDS on households will be felt on income, productivity, consumption, employment, health and non-health expenditures, schooling of children, and the health of other family members.[75] Recounting the example of Thailand, Indrani Gupta says that 'one-third of rural families experienced a halving of their agricultural output, and another 15 per cent had to withdraw their children from the school due to the disease'.[76] It has been abundantly observed in many families that as adults fall sick and die, households feel the effects of the loss of adult farm labour, which leads to a sharp decline in productivity, loss of income, and increase in household expenditures. Ashok Rao says that this is clearly evident today in Karnataka, as many of his patients are from the agriculture belt of northern Karnataka where farmers have small landholdings. He says that it is already evident how farmers' inability to work on their farms is affecting agricultural output.[77] A World Bank study shows that households in India spend between 5 and 7 per cent of their income on health. And rural households spend even more, that is, 12–19 per cent. HIV/AIDS will, in all likelihood, sharply increase this expenditure.[78]

According to UNAIDS, when a family member is infected with

[74] Ekstrand et al., 'HIV/AIDS in India', p. 54.
[75] Indrani Gupta, 'Do we still need more evidence?', p. 23.
[76] Ibid.
[77] Interview with Ashok Rao.
[78] Ekstrand et al., 'HIV/AIDS in India', p. 108.

HIV, household income can decline by as much as 40 to 60 per cent because the sick become less productive, subsequent death results in loss of income, and, in most cases, family members leave their jobs to take care of the HIV-infected members.[79]

Even if there is a cure for AIDS, this situation is unlikely to radically change as poor households would not be able to buy the drugs, and the government may not be willing to spend for all victims. As Ajay Mahal says, in the long run, members of households affected by HIV/AIDS will have lower accumulations of human capital in education or health.[80] This scenario is likely to perpetuate the misery of the affected household as there is hardly any social security net which can take care of the HIV/AIDS infected.

A study by Indrani Gupta which looked at the economic impact on HIV-positive individuals showed that the group on an average spent between 10 to 30 per cent of their annual income on HIV-related expenditures, most of which was on drugs and medicines.[81] Households will not only have to spend for HIV-related medicines but also on opportunistic disease expenses, which also can be very huge.

A survey was conducted in the Sangli district of Maharashtra, to assess the impact of an adult HIV/AIDS-related death on the household in general and children in particular. Three types of households were taken up for the study which had a total of 118 households with an HIV/AIDS death, 100 households with a non-HIV/AIDS-related death and 100 households with no deaths. Households with HIV/AIDS deaths reported reduced savings during the period of observation, reduced expenditures on consumer durable items, and disposal of assets in order to raise or supplement income. There were instances of discrimination against them and some of them had to send their children away to relatives or withdraw them from school. An adult member infected with HIV meant children being denied education and health care.[82]

[79] 'HIV/AIDS as a Security Issue', ICG report, p. 6.

[80] Mahal, 'Economic implications of inertia on HIV/AIDS and Benefits of Action', p. 1052.

[81] Indrani Gupta et al., 'HIV/AIDS and Development in India', p. 13.

[82] Ravi K. Verma et al., 'HIV/AIDS and children in the Sangli district of Maharashtra', in Giovanni Andrea Cornia (ed.), *AIDS, Public Policy and Child*

India's intercity goods transport sector could also be at risk in the days to come. Intercity truckers amounting to some 3–5 million are understood to be a high-risk category, both in acquiring and in transmitting HIV. Estimates say that the number of truck drivers contracting HIV increases at the rate of 1,000 truckers every week.[83] According to a survey of truck drivers in 2000, the proportion of respondents who reported having sex with any kind of partner (married or other partners) during the preceding year (1999) ranged between 92 per cent among truck drivers and 64 per cent among truck helpers.[84] The percentage of truck drivers who had sex with FSWS was 36, and it was 47 among truck helpers. Besides 12 per cent of truck drivers had sex with non-regular partners as the percentage among truck helpers was 23. Moreover, 22 per cent of truck drivers, 28 per cent truck helpers and 45 per cent of stationary workers had reported having had one commercial partner during the preceding year. While the survey results do not say what this behaviour pattern will mean *vis-à-vis* the spread of HIV/AIDS among this group, one may be right in considering that at least some of them had not used a condom and thus may have contracted HIV/AIDS. Moreover, this survey captures only a small fraction of India's national highway network of 52,000 km. spanning 35 states, on which thousands of truckers ply everyday.

In a set of 2000–1 STI/HIV-prevalence surveys conducted among male truckers in West Bengal (East), Andhra Pradesh (South), and Haryana (North), it was found that in eastern India, the prevalence of HIV was 2.99 per cent, syphilis 6.3 per cent and gonorrhea 1.8 per cent. In the north, the prevalence of HIV among associations-based truckers was 1.9 per cent, while syphilis and

---

Well-Being, available at http://www.unicef-icdc.org/research/ESP/aids/chapter8.pdf.

[83] These figures were given by the Department of International Development (DFID), London as part of a Project Memorandum in 1996. Copy of the Memorandum is available at http://www.unescap. org/tctd/pubs/hiv01_2_6.htm.

[84] 'Summary Report: Behavioural Surveillance Survey in Healthy Highway Project, India: Part 4', Family Health International, 2001, available at http://www.fhi.org/en/HIVAIDS/pub/survreports/BSSHealthyHwy/BSSHealthyHwy4.htm.

gonorrhea were 7.2 and 4.8 per cent respectively. The prevalence of HIV and syphilis was higher among truckers from halt points in the north—HIV 6.9 per cent, syphilis 8.4 per cent. However, in south India, the prevalence of HIV was 10.9 per cent, while syphilis and gonorrhea were 9.6 per cent and 7.5 per cent respectively. Also 27 per cent of truckers from the east, 49.4 per cent from the south, 29 per cent of association–based truckers and 45.3 per cent of truckers from halt points from the north reported having sex with female sex workers in the preceding year. The percentage of reported condom use during the last sex encounter with FSW/NRP was 30.4 per cent in the east, 57.2 per cent in the south, and 16.6 per cent among association-based and 12 per cent among halt point-based truckers in the north.[85]

It is true that many of these truck workers are easily replaceable, at least for some time to come, if they contract HIV/AIDS and fall ill, and hence will not really affect India's goods transport sector in a major way in the years to come. However, such replaceability is certainly not going to be a permanent feature, and what it will mean to a country's economy if thousands of truckers are going to be infected with HIV/AIDS has been dealt with in detail in the previous section.

Diminishing efficiency and productivity at places of work due to HIV/AIDS is a problem that many African countries are facing today. India, though not on a very large scale, is also increasingly facing this problem.

Many people may think that to consider HIV/AIDS as having a negative impact on India's economy is a wild exaggeration. The following examples which show how diseases in the past have affected trade and economy will help them to see true position.

1. Malaria in Africa: The WHO estimates that Africa's GDP would be nearly $100 billion greater if malaria had been eliminated 35 years ago.[86]
2. Avian flu in Hong Kong: The avian influenza outbreak in 1997

[85] Ekstrand et al., 'HIV/AIDS in India', p. 56.

[86] Barbara Boxer, 'Providing Basic Human Security', *The Washington Quarterly*, Spring 2003, p. 202, available at www.twq.com/03spring/docs/03spring_boxer.pdf.

cost the former colony hundreds of millions of dollars in lost poultry production, commerce, and tourism, with airport arrivals in November of that year alone down by 22 per cent from the preceding year.

3. Bovine spongiform encephalopathy (BSE) and New variant Creutzfeldt-Jakob Disease (nvCJD) in Britain: The outbreak of BSE and new variant Creutzfeldt-Jakob disease in the United Kingdom in 1995 prompted a mass slaughter of cattle, cut beef consumption drastically, and led to the imposition of a three-year EU embargo against British beef. The losses to the British economy were estimated by the WHO at $5.75 billion including $2 billion in lost beef exports.
4. Cyclospora in Guatemalan raspberries: The outbreak of cyclospora-related illness in the United States and Canada associated with raspberries from Guatemala led to curbs in imports that cost Guatemala several million dollars in lost revenue.
5. Cholera in Peru: The outbreak of cholera in 1991 cost the Peruvian fishing industry an estimated $775 million in lost tourism and trade because of a temporary ban on seafood exports.
6. Foot and mouth disease in Taiwan: In 1997, an outbreak of foot and mouth disease (FMD) devastated Taiwan's pork industry—one of the largest in the world—shutting down exports for a full year.
7. Nipah in Malaysia: In 1999, the Nipah virus caused the shutdown of over half of the country's pig farms and an embargo against pork exports.
8. Plague in India: The plague outbreak in Surat, India, in 1994 and the ensuing panic sparked a sudden exodus of 0.5 million people from the region and led to abrupt shutdowns of entire industries, including aviation and tourism, as several countries froze trade, banned travel from India, and sent some Indian migrants home. The WHO estimated the outbreak cost India some $2 billion.[87]

[87] Gannon, 'The Global Infectious Diseases Threat and its Implications for the United States', January 2000, available at http://www.cia.gov/cia/reports/nie/report/nie99-17d.html.

HIV/AIDS AS A SOCIETAL SECURITY THREAT

Societal security may be understood as the relative preservation of a society's time-honoured structures, time-tested institutions and the well-being of its members. HIV/AIDS has the capacity to destroy these very members of the society and their institutions. The World Bank makes the picture clear when it says:

> First, AIDS selectively destroys human capital, that is, peoples' accumulated life experiences, their human and job skills, and their knowledge and insights built up over a period of years. It is primarily a disease of young adults. As these infected adults become progressively sick and weak, they steadily lose their ability to work. Eventually, the disease kills them in their prime, thereby destroying the human capital built up in them over the years through child-rearing, formal education, and learning on the job.
>
> Second, AIDS weakens or even wrecks the mechanisms that generate human capital formation. In family homes, the quality of child-rearing depends heavily on the parents' human capital. If one or, worse, both parents die while their children are still young, the transmission of knowledge and potential productive capacity across the two generations will be weakened. At the same time, the loss of income due to disability and early death reduces the lifetime resources available to the family, which may well result in the children spending much less time (if any at all) at school.
>
> Third, the chance that the children themselves will contract the disease in adulthood makes investment in their education less attractive, even when both parents themselves remain uninfected. Thus with too little education and knowledge gathered from their parents, as well as being deprived of parental love and guidance throughout their childhood, the children of AIDS victims later become adults who themselves are less able to raise their own children and to invest in their education. The process is insidious, since the effects are felt only over the long run, as the poor education of children today translates into low adult productivity a generation later, and so on. But if nothing is done, the report warns, the outbreak of the disease will eventually precipitate economic collapse.[88]

There are other ways in which HIV/AIDS can produce social

[88] 'Economic costs of AIDS', World Bank Group, 23 July 2003. Available at http://www.globalpolicy.org/socecon/develop/2003/0723costs.htm.

instability. HIV/AIDS would, in course of time, as Richard Holbrooke argues, create a unique, new untouchable caste, the existence of which could provoke violence and civil strife.[89] It will disturb communal harmony, create inter-regional discords, and produce AIDS orphans who, in turn, would threaten societal security at large. An AIDS pandemic could also lead to a growing number of people becoming disengaged from their societies and seeking alternative and even violent ways of securing their livelihood.[90] The sub-Saharan African experience of having to live with HIV/AIDS tells us that where an AIDS crisis is severe, governing institutions and civil society are already weak or threatened. In a recent study, Peter Gordon, Ruth Jacobson, and Tom Porteous point out that while in countries like India, China, and Russia overall political stability may not be affected by HIV/AIDS as 'the much larger populations of states like China, Russia and India will be better able to absorb the economic and social impacts of the disease, and because their governments are more capable of responding effectively to the disease', it is possible that localized violence may 'occur in these countries due to perceptions that governments are failing to address the issue of HIV/AIDS (there has already been unrest in China) or due to manipulation of perceptions and prejudices about HIV/AIDS.'[91]

Migration-related HIV/AIDS infections are likely to create problems and irritants among different regions of the country. Former Punjab Health Minister Baldev Raj Chawla has gone on record to say that migrants from other states are the biggest health threat to the state, because he thinks, they bring contagious diseases like AIDS.[92] Orissa's Ganjam district benefits greatly from its people who work in Gujarat—around 9 lakhs of them—and bring cash

[89] Elbe, 'Strategic implications of HIV/AIDS', p. 56.

[90] Ibid.

[91] Peter Gordon, Ruth Jacobson and Tom Porteous, 'A Study to Establish the Connections Between Hiv/Aids & Conflict', February 2004, available at http://www.jsiuk.com/docs/hiv_aids_conflict_2004.pdf.

[92] 'Punjab minister calls migrants a health threat', *Indian Express*, New Delhi, 4 December 2001, available at http://www.indianexpress.com/ie20011204/nat6.html.

and AIDS back into the state. We may want to remind ourselves about the 'anti-Bihari' riots that took place in Assam in 2004. AIDS could be a cause for such tensions. Within a state it is likely that certain highly HIV/AIDS infected areas may be shunned by other regions. Social relations like marriage may be affected. One example would be the Namakkal district of Tamil Nadu which has one of India's highest rates of HIV/AIDS after the Sangli district of Maharashtra.

As pointed out earlier marriage is one such sacred institution that could be at risk in the days to come. Indrani Gupta et al., note that in states like Tamil Nadu marriage itself is a risk factor for many Indian women who might contract the disease through marriage. They cite a study which reported an HIV-prevalence rate of 4 per cent in a rural setting.[93] If in today's Indian marriage system factors like caste, star sign, and dowry do matter, HIV status might also become an important factor. Andhra Pradesh is already contemplating legislation making HIV testing mandatory before marriage.[94]

With HIV/AIDS attempting to and succeeding in destroying the primary unit of what constitutes a nation, the family, one section of society which is at acute risk today is children—AIDS orphans, more precisely. India currently has around 12.6 lakhs AIDS orphans, a figure which is likely to double in just a few years and will be 25 lakhs by 2010.[95] A World Bank study rightly points out that:

> The impacts of the AIDS crisis have not begun to emerge fully in India, and AIDS-related orphaning is not yet occurring at a large scale. Yet, India has the largest number of AIDS orphans of any country in the

[93] Indrani Gupta et al., 'HIV/AIDS and Development in India', p. 10.

[94] 'HIV prevention: Should there be compulsory screening?', *BBC Online*, 29 November 2002, available at http://news.bbc.co.uk/1/hi/talking_point/debates/south_asian/2511103.stm. Also see, 'K'taka intends law for compulsory HIV test before wedding', *Hindustan Times*, New Delhi, 2 August 2004, available at http://www.hindustantimes.com/2004/Aug/02/181_924562,000900020002.htm.

[95] Subhadra Menon, 'India's Widening AIDS Epidemic', *BBC Online*, 28 November 2003, available at http://news.bbc.co.uk/2/hi/south_asia/3250285.stm.

world. This number is expected to more than double in five years, and the proportion of orphaned children will remain exceptionally high until 2020 or 2030. Given the long incubation period between infection and the onset of symptoms, the epidemic's impact will linger for decades even if the rate of new infections is brought under control.[96]

A study of children in 10 Indian cities demonstrates that the number of children on the streets will rise more rapidly in the years ahead as HIV/AIDS takes away parents from children. These children, if they do not already have HIV/AIDS, are highly vulnerable to contracting HIV/AIDS and would be further marginalized in society. The Calcutta Samaritans, an organization that takes care of orphans, estimates that over 1 lakh children on the city's streets have almost no education and few life or vocational skills.[97]

In India, which has the world's largest number of AIDS orphans, the number is on the increase as out of the 27 million deliveries that take place every year, 1.3 lakhs occur in mothers who are HIV-positive.[98]

If only one parent of the child dies, he or she is often withdrawn from school to help increase the family income or, in the case of girls, to take charge of the younger children. It is not a long before these children lose both parents. They then experience social stigma, discrimination, isolation, vulnerability, depression, fear, lack of access to education and health care, malnutrition, and homelessness.[99] Many a time they are denied access to schooling, health care, inheritance rights, etc.

[96] http://www1.worldbank.org/sp/safetynets/OVCWorkshop_5-03/Handout_India.pdf

[97] K.M. Misra, et al. 'Primary prevention programme amongst street and working children—a pioneering collaborative effort between a NGO and a University,' XIV International Conference on AIDS, Barcelona, 7–12 July 2002, cited in Ekstrand et al., p. 110.

[98] A World Bank report reveals that India has the largest number of AIDS orphans. See 'At-a-Glance – India: AIDS and orphans', Vasavya Mahila Mandli, available at http://www1.worldbank.org/sp/safetynets/OVCWorkshop_5-03/Handout_India.pdf. A report in *The Hindustan Times* suggested that the number of AIDS orphans is on the rise. See '10 per cent of AIDS affected are children', *Hindustan Times*, New Delhi, 6 November 2001.

[99] A.C.V. Arumugam, 'Challenges faced by caa of rural area of theni dt.,tamil

Most of these children, shunned by society and relatives and bearing the stigma of a horrible disease, become social outcasts and are usually left to roam the streets on the fringes of society, more often engaging in petty crime and prostitution, either contracting HIV/AIDS or giving it to others. More often than not the families are dissolved in course of time. One study in Zambia found that 55 per cent of the households in which the mother had died had dissolved.[100]

Ekstrand et al., rightly point out that 'child vulnerability is already high in India with large numbers of orphans and displaced children, a growing number of street children, poor quality or over burdened child welfare institutions, and wide scale abuse and exploitation of children.'[101] Such children, often considered social outcasts, are easy to indoctrinate and to get to do wrong things. There is no dearth of crime, insurgencies and subversive activities in India, and these AIDS orphans, who will grow up impoverished and mostly uneducated, prone to criminal behaviour and disenchanted with society, will be easily recruited for such criminal activities. Such threats are even more likely in a society like India, where there are large economic disparities and very few opportunities, even for those not HIV-positive. Organized crime in Mumbai, for example, can provide the basic amenities and thus meaning to many of these youngsters. Moreover, at the height of any epidemic, crime rates go up. For example, during the plague epidemics in India between 1896 and 1914, crime rates had reportedly increased considerably.[102] AIDS will only make any such crisis situation graver.

An AIDS orphan may thus be considered to be a child soldier in the making, to fight wars for his or her existence, the difference being that an AIDS orphan, unlike in a real war, is not disciplined, not trained, not paid and not given a specific enemy: society is his/her enemy.

nadu.-pwds-alliance project experience', XIV International Conference on AIDS, Barcelona, 7-12 July 2002, cited in Ekstrand et al., p. 110.

[100] 'HIV/AIDS as a Security Issue', ICG Report, p. 6.

[101] Ekstrand et al., 'HIV/AIDS in India', p. 12.

[102] Elbe, 'Strategic implications of HIV/AIDS', p. 57.

CONCLUSION

The first section of this chapter has argued that if human security is about the protection from direct and indirect threats to the personal safety and well-being of the individual, then HIV/AIDS constitutes a human security threat. In a nutshell, this section has argued that HIV/AIDS destroys human security both at the individual and at the collective level because it causes individual suffering and death, HIV/AIDS victims contact other opportunistic diseases, fall prey to the normal Indian practice of making them social outcasts, it kills people at an extremely productive and reproductive age, and creates demographic problems within the country. This human suffering, which goes on to destroy a considerable proportion of a state's population constitutes a direct threat to that state's security.

The second section has argued that HIV/AIDS is also a threat to India's economic security. While there is just not enough data to generate figures as to what will be the economic fallout of the disease in India, the available data, albeit partial, itself suggests that the country will lose billions of dollars due to AIDS. Studies have also not been able to capture the exact nature of the losses that will adversely affect India's economy. Various sectoral studies conducted in different parts of the country have indicated that the disease will affect the national economy in GDP terms, the health sector, industry, transport sector, labour productivity, foreign trade, household income, etc. The third section of the chapter has argued that HIV/AIDS can also prove to be a traditional security threat to India. First, Indian military and paramilitary forces operating in difficult circumstances in Jammu & Kashmir and the north-east, having been away from home for long periods of time are likely to contract the disease on a large scale. This could affect the national security interests of the country including peacekeeping operations and power projection. Police forces in cities like Mumbai, Pune, Bangalore and Chennai are also contracting the disease. HIV/AIDS also has the potential to raise cross-border problems.

The final section in this chapter has argued that the societal security of the country, understood as the relative preservation of a society's time-honoured structures, time-tested institutions and the well-being of its members, can also be jeopardized by the disease. People can be disengaged from their societies, AIDS orphans can take to criminal activities, intergovernmental discords can take place, and social institutions like marriage can lose their present shape and form due to HIV/AIDS, leading to social instability and chaos.

CHAPTER 3

Three Dangerous Factors: Poverty, Ignorance and Stigma

This chapter will analyze how poverty, ignorance, and the social stigma attached to the disease can prove to be accelerators of the epidemic in the country. Many developed Western countries are also facing the problem of HIV/AIDS. HIV/AIDS could, however, become a security threat, particularly for a country like India because of three factors: poverty, ignorance about the disease, and the widespread social stigma attached to it. Whereas one factor itself or in combination with the disease can be dangerous, India, unfortunately, is faced with the interplay of all these three factors. This chapter will first look at poverty and AIDS, then at ignorance and AIDS, and finally, stigma and AIDS.

POVERTY AND AIDS

There is no doubt that widespread abject poverty is a fact of life in India. The Indian government has, of late, been refining and redefining the methodology used to measure the incidence of poverty in India. In 1999–2000, around 27.09 per cent of India's rural population and around 23.62 per cent of its urban population was living in poverty.[1] What is being talked about here is crores of Indians. According to the World Bank, for the year 2000, 28.6 per cent of the Indian people were living below the poverty line.[2] Poverty increases the instance of HIV/AIDS and also its deadly

[1] Indrani Gupta et al., 'HIV/AIDS and Development in India', p. 9.

[2] 'The HIV/AIDS crisis in India', *South Asia Monitor*, CSIS, 1 May 2003, p. 1, available at www.csis.org/saprog/sam58.pdf.

nature. While malnutrition and lack of health care can kill HIV-positive people faster, poverty prompts people to take to professions like sex work which increases the incidence of HIV/AIDS. HIV/AIDS specifically targets the poor for the simple reason that the poor households bear a much greater economic burden due to infections than their wealthier counterparts.[3]

Hakan Björkman, an adviser on HIV/AIDS to UNDP's Bureau for Development Policy, states that:

> HIV/AIDS is not strictly speaking a disease of poverty as it affects people at all income levels. But evidence from some countries at advanced states of the epidemic shows that new HIV infections disproportionately affect poor people, unskilled workers, and those lacking literacy skills especially young women in each of these categories. The relationship among poverty, gender, and HIV vulnerability has important policy implications.[4]

A brief glance at the country's poor would help us understand why poverty and AIDS is such a deadly combination. Seasonally employed people, informal sector workers, street children, beggars, slum dwellers, sex workers, most of those who are illiterate or uneducated, the marginalized and disempowered, refugees, and sexual minorities normally live below the poverty line. These people are likely to sell sex to make a living or visit a female sex worker for occasional entertainment as many of them do not live with a family and would not be able to visit a doctor if they were infected by HIV/AIDS.

Twenty nine per cent of Indians, mostly poor, use public health facilities when they fall ill.[5] The condition of India's public hospitals needs no description. More often than not there is no doctor, or medicine, or facilities for inpatient treatment. Only 10 per cent of Indians have health insurance, leaving the rest to fend for themselves.[6] In such circumstances, many prefer to live with the sickness, and thereby spread it, rather than spend any money to go

[3] Price-Smith, 'Pretoria's Shadow', p. 9.

[4] Björkman, 'HIV/AIDS and Poverty Reduction Strategies', UNDP Policy Note, New York: UNDP, Bureau for Development Policy, 2002, cited in Ekstrand et al., p. 41.

[5] Ibid., p. 65.

[6] Ibid.

to private clinics: most often they simply do not have a choice. The poor also reportedly sell their blood to earn a living, most often transmitting deadly diseases including HIV with the blood.

IGNORANCE AND AIDS

Ignorance can make HIV/AIDS deadlier due to three reasons: first, nine out of ten people infected do not know they are HIV-positive and are likely to go on spreading the infection;[7] second, those not infected are not aware of the disease and may engage in risky behaviour; and third, the general public, due to lack of knowledge again, may not take HIV/AIDS prevention programmes kindly as has been increasingly seen in many parts of the country.

India's National Baseline Behaviour Surveillance Survey (BSS) mentions that overall awareness of HIV/AIDS in India is 76 per cent. While 82 per cent of men were aware of HIV/AIDS, the figure for women was 70 per cent. Nearly 7 per cent of adults, the survey says, reported having sex with a non-regular partner in the last 12 months. Only 33 per cent of these respondents reported consistent condom use with all non-regular partners.[8] Fifty per cent of sex workers reported consistent condom use with paying clients in the last 30 days. However, among those who had had non-paying partners in the 3 months prior to the survey, only 21 per cent reported using condoms consistently.[9]

The above official survey data shows that awareness about how unprotected sex leads to contracting infections like HIV/AIDS is very low in the general public. It may also be necessary to look at the extent of premarital sex and the risks associated with it. A study conducted by the National Institute of Health and Family Welfare and coordinated by V.K. Tiwari, says that a quarter to a third of India's young people indulge in premarital sex. The study 'surveyed premarital sex and unmet contraceptive needs among school children and college students, young working men and

[7] 'Isabelle Claxton, 'The right to know', Seminar–520, December 2002, p. 45.

[8] National Baseline General Population Behavioural Surveillance Survey, 2001, New Delhi, available at http://www.naco.nic.in/nacp/publctn.htm.

[9] Ibid.

women, and young people aged 15 to 24 years living in slums in Delhi and Lucknow'.[10] The conclusion of the study is that the premarital sex rate varies from 17 per cent among school-children to 33 per cent among young workers in the typical North Indian population. The study also demolishes the myth that metropolitan cities have a greater incidence of premarital sex than other cities. The study says that premarital sex was more common in Lucknow than in Delhi.[11] It would be foolish to suppose that all college-going or working men and women who indulge in premarital sex would do it protected.[12] Dr Ashok Rao notes that most people do not think a healthy looking sex worker can have HIV/AIDS.[13]

Around 75 per cent of women in the rural areas of Bihar, Gujarat and UP have never heard of HIV/AIDS.[14] A study of the migrants in Delhi showed that 56 per cent of the sample had not even heard of the disease. Lack of awareness sometimes goes in the other direction. One survey shows that more than 60 per cent of Indians mistakenly believe that they can contract AIDS from mosquito bites or by sharing a meal or shaking hands with an HIV-infected person.[15] The Helping Hand Foundation and the Bihar State AIDS Control Society conducted a study in Gaya's red-light areas and came to the conclusion that 80 per cent of the sex workers in Gaya are unaware of HIV/AIDS.[16]

Ignorance becomes even more dangerous when women are ignorant because, though not knowingly, it is women who play a big role in transmitting the disease to others or to their children. Awareness of AIDS among women has increased but it is still

[10] Rohit Sharma, 'More than a quarter of India's youngsters have pre-marital sex', *British Medical Journal*, 10 March 2001, available at www.bmj.com/cgi/collection/AIDS.

[11] Ibid.

[12] 'AIDS cases up by 610,000', *Business Standard*, New Delhi, 14 November 2003.

[13] Interview with Ashok Rao.

[14] 'AIDS cases up by 610,000', *Business Standard*.

[15] Schaffer et al., 'India at the crossroads', p. 8.

[16] Arun Srivastava, 'AIDS unknown to sex workers in Gaya: Study', *Indian Express*, 21 May 2001, available at http://www.indianexpress.com/ie20010521/nat7.html.

quite low—around 40 per cent nationwide. One-third of women who have heard of it do not know the ways to avoid it.[17] It is reported that despite knowing that their partners are HIV-positive, Indian women engage in unprotected sex with them due to limited access to contraceptive methods such as female condoms, microbicides and because of the social inequalities that promote the subordination of women.[18] According to one survey, 46 per cent of women never used condoms, 22 per cent used them sometimes, and 17 per cent always used them.[19] The survey also indicated that while some people have heard of HIV/AIDS, awareness of how to prevent infection is low. Nearly all respondents in four community-based studies on gender and HIV/AIDS sponsored by the United Nations Development Fund for Women (UNIFEM) in 2000, said that the condom was primarily for contraception.[20] While almost 50 per cent of sex workers in sensitized sites are HIV-positive, only 57 per cent of the clients of female sex workers reported consistent condom use as per the behavioural surveillance survey in 2001.[21] This was confirmed (to this author) by sex workers in Mumbai and Pune. They stated that if they insist that clients use a condom, the clients shun them thinking that they actually have some infection. Moreover, very often a large number of the condoms distributed among sex workers are sold by them to earn petty cash.[22] See Figure 3.1 to understand what percentage of men use condoms while having sex with non-regular partners.

[17] 'Women are becoming increasingly affected by HIV', *The Pioneer*, New Delhi, 8 March 2002.

[18] Sambamoorthi et al., 'Antenatal care and AIDS knowledge among married women', p. 723.

[19] Rohit Sharma, 'More than a quarter of India's youngsters have pre-marital sex'.

[20] Ann Ninan, 'Without my consent: Women and HIV-related stigma in India', available at www.prb.org/Template.cfm?Section=PRB&template=/ContentManagement/ContentDisplay.cfm&ContentID=8278.

[21] 'AIDS cases up by 610,000', *Business Standard*.

[22] Interview with Ashok Rao.

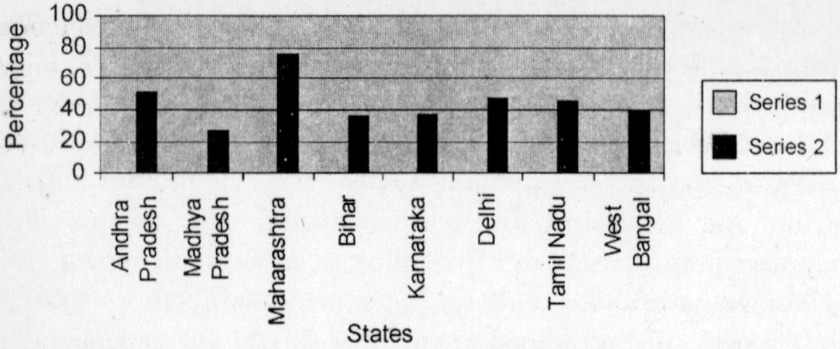

Source: Behavioural Surveillance Survey, India, 2001[23]

FIGURE 3.1: PERCENTAGE OF MALES REPORTING CONDOM USE WITH LAST NON-REGULAR PARTNER IN THE PAST YEAR, 2001

STIGMA AND AIDS

Widespread social stigma in India is the third factor which makes HIV/AIDS very dangerous. Repercussions of the widespread stigma operate at many levels—from villages to offices in India's metropolitan cities. It contributes to the suffering of those infected and their relatives, interferes with decision making on HIV counselling and testing one's HIV status, and seeking and remaining in prolonged treatment.[24] Attacks against AIDS patients are not uncommon in the country. The scene is worse in the interior villages where ignorance and myths about the disease are the order of the day. Villagers do not want to talk about the disease, let alone take blood tests. If a person in a community develops the disease, he/she faces complete social expulsion. In many parts of India, AIDS patients live no better than animals.[25] Vijay Nair, head of the Mumbai-based UDDAN Trust, an NGO working for HIV-positive homosexual men, says that in most cases students are expelled from schools.[26]

[23] Behavioural Surveillance Survey, India, 2001.

[24] Ekstrand et al., 'HIV/AIDS in India', p. 71.

[25] Mohuya Choudhuri, 'Indian Migrant Workers: Sweatshop conditions/ ignorance lead to AIDS epidemic', available at http://www.comminit.com/ Commentary/sld-4103.html.

[26] Interview with Vijay Nair in Mumbai on 2 February 2004.

Dr Shalini Bharat of the Tata Institute of Social Sciences, Mumbai, in her study on HIV/AIDS-related discrimination, stigma and denial in Bangalore and Mumbai, talks extensively about the main overt and covert forms of discriminations faced by HIV/AIDS patients. They are:[27]

General

- Physical isolation at home (e.g. separate sleeping arrangements)
- Blocked entry to common areas or facilities (toilet, etc.)
- Blocked entry to common places like village or a neighbourhood area
- Denial of death rituals
- Labelling and name-calling

Workplace

- Removal from job
- Forced resignation
- Withdrawal of health/insurance benefits
- Poor access to shared facilities
- Social distance
- Labelling and name-calling

There were also more covert forms of stigma in these sites.

Hospitals

- Delays in treatment; slow service (e.g. made to wait in queues, asked to come again)
- Excuses or explanations given for non-admission (but admission not directly refused)
- Shunting patient between wards/doctors/hospitals
- Keeping patient under observation without any treatment plan

[27] Shalini Bharat, 'India: HIV and AIDS-related Discrimination, Stigmatization and Denial', August 2001, pp. 16–17, available at www.thebody.com/unaids/pdfs/india.pdf.

- Postponed treatment or operations
- Unnecessarily repeating HIV tests
- Conditional treatment (e.g. only on the condition that the patient will come for follow-up or join a drug trial programme).

Home and Community

- Disparaging remarks about the HIV-positive family member (e.g. 'he is paying for past sins')
- 'Guilt tripping' for burdening the family economy and for lowering family prestige

During the survey mentioned earlier, conducted in the Sangli district in Maharashtra, many respondents recall discrimination whereby they had to send their children away to distant relatives or withdraw them from school.[28]

CONCLUSION

The first section has argued that widespread poverty in India, amounting to around 25 per cent nationwide, can increase HIV/AIDS through malnutrition, poverty-induced sex trade/prostitution or sell contaminated blood risking the further spread of the disease; and due to the lack of access to health care.

The second section has argued that ignorance can make HIV/AIDS deadlier, for the following reasons: first, nine out of ten people infected do not know they are HIV-positive and are likely to go on spreading it; second, those not infected are not aware of the disease and may engage in risky behaviour; and third, the general public, due to lack of knowledge again, may not take HIV/AIDS prevention programmes kindly as has been increasingly seen in many parts of the country.

The final section of the chapter has argued that the widespread stigma about HIV/AIDS as prevalent in the country can make it

[28] Ravi K. Verma et al., 'HIV/AIDS and children in the Sangli district of Maharashtra', p. 1.

very dangerous as it contributes to the suffering of those infected and their relatives, interferes with decision-making on HIV counselling and on testing one's HIV status, and seeking and remaining in prolonged treatment.

CHAPTER 4

The Experiences of Other Regions/Countries

This chapter attempts to briefly describe the HIV/AIDS situation in Africa, and more specifically in South Africa. It also includes a section on the success of the anti-AIDS campaign in Thailand. The first section will deal with the African experience in general, followed by sections on South Africa and Thailand.

HIV/AIDS: THE AFRICAN EXPERIENCE

The sub-Saharan experience of dealing with or suffering the impact of HIV/AIDS must be understood for the following reasons. First, the African experience will tell us how a disease over the years has become a security threat of immense proportions, threatening the very existence of many of those countries; second, in many respects what is happening in Africa is perhaps an indication of what may happen in many countries of Asia, Eastern Europe and the Caribbean;[1] third, it can tell us what could happen if we do not learn from the experiences of others; and finally, there is a lot in common between how HIV/AIDS became a security threat there and the way it is becoming one in India.

A common 'syndrome' in most of the HIV/AIDS-affected African countries is millions of people waiting to die, hundreds of thousands of AIDS orphans, industrial productivity taking a nosedive, factories shutting down due to the shortage of workers, etc. A study by USAID of specific African countries reached the

[1] Mark Schneider and Michael Moodie, 'The destabilizing impacts of HIV/AIDS', May 2002, p. 4, available at http://www.csis.org/africa/0205_DestImp.pdf.

conclusion that a 2.6 per cent annual decline in GDP occurs for countries with infection rates above 20 per cent.[2] A study on Namibia showed that AIDS cost the country nearly 8 per cent of GDP in 1996, while a study of Kenya projected that its GDP will be 14.5 per cent smaller in 2005 than it would otherwise have been without the cumulative impact of AIDS.[3] The Food and Agriculture Organization (FAO) estimates that since 1985, 7 million agricultural workers have died from AIDS-related diseases in 27 African countries. In the hardest hit countries, the study claims, AIDS has killed almost 13 per cent of the agricultural workforce, or one in seven workers, and another 16 million will die in the next two decades, accounting for 26 per cent of the labour force in the most affected African countries.[4]

In many African countries, the slackening of economic growth is already intensifying the competition between economic and political elites for the resources available in the country resulting in political violence, misgovernance, coups, etc. HIV/AIDS will add to this problem, if it is not already doing it.

International investors and businessmen are already shunning the African countries. A study by a British House of Commons committee reported evidence of investment moving out of Africa. The study talks about 50 individual companies determining that HIV/AIDS would substantially affect their potential regional market and that they were better off investing elsewhere.[5] It is understandable why MNCs would not want to invest in sub-Saharan African countries where it is reported that companies are hiring two or three workers for a single worker's job because one or two are expected to die from HIV/AIDS.[6]

There is going to be a critical demographic change in many African countries: estimates say that 19 of the 27 countries where children will lose one or both parents to AIDS by 2010 are in

[2] Ibid.

[3] Gannon, 'The Global Infectious Diseases Threat and its Implications for the United States'.

[4] 'HIV/AIDS as a Security Issue', ICG Report, p. 11.

[5] Ibid.

[6] Boxer, 'Providing Basic Human Security', p. 202.

sub-Saharan Africa.[7] HIV/AIDS is eating into the educational edifice of the African countries as, on the one hand, teachers are falling prey to the disease, and on the other, students are increasingly being pulled out from school. 'In sub-Saharan Africa in 1999, 860,000 primary school children lost their teachers to AIDS. Africa is expected to lose 10 per cent of its teachers to AIDS by 2005, setting back education levels by 100 years, according to the USAID.'[8]

HIV/AIDS is also not leaving governance in the affected countries untouched. Reports indicate that in Africa, civil servants, especially security personnel, suffer from higher rates of HIV infection than the general population.[9] The military is probably the worst sufferer. According to the estimates of the US Defense Intelligence Agency, 40–60 per cent of the soldiers in Angola's army and 70–5 per cent of the personnel in Zimbabwe's and Malawi's armies are HIV-positive.[10]

SOUTH AFRICA: THE TRIUMPH OF HIV/AIDS

With more than 4.7 million South Africans infected with HIV and prevalence rates of 20 per cent in the adult population, South Africa, which has seen 1,700 or so new contractions every day, is on the verge of surrendering to HIV/AIDS.[11] What is threatened is not South Africa's national security, but its national existence.

As per the estimates given by the US Bureau of the Census, nearly 25 per cent of the total South African population will be HIV-positive by 2010. In addition, more than 50 per cent of those are in the range of 30 to 35 years, and more than 8 million South Africans will have died from the disease. Life expectancy will come

[7] Gannon, 'The Global Infectious Diseases Threat and its Implications for the United States'.

[8] 'HIV/AIDS as a National Security Issue', ICG Report.

[9] 'The Destabilizing Impact of HIV/AIDS', CSIS, 2002, p. 6, available at http://www.csis.org/africa/0205_DestImp.pdf.

[10] Ibid.

[11] Price-Smith, 'Pretoria's Shadow', p. 4.

down to a depressing 35 years.[12] The South African Health Minister, T Shabalala-misuin, has gone on record to say that AIDS deaths in South Africa in 2004 would be 4 lakhs per year, and 5 lakhs in 2010.[13] The last decade has been most crucial for the country as it saw a tragic increase in infection levels, which rose from 1 per cent in 1990 to 25 per cent of the South African population in 2000.[14]

A World Bank report claims that in South Africa, GDP will be 17 per cent lower by 2010 than it would have been without the AIDS epidemic.[15] Studies have mentioned that 'over the next 10 years the disease could reduce South Africa's gross domestic product (GDP) by 17 per cent and take away $22,000 million from the national economy'.[16] Andrew Price-Smith says, 'the average annual growth rate will decline by .1 per cent (from 2002–5), 0.3 per cent (2006–10) and by .9 per cent (2011–15).'[17] Moreover, HIV/AIDS is likely to reduce investor confidence in the country, leading to capital flight from the country.

In many of South Africa's industries, large chunks of the work-force are HIV-positive. Lonmins, a major firm that produces platinum, has recently estimated that more than 26 per cent of its workforce is now HIV-positive.[18] A survey in a gold-mining area near Johannesburg revealed that, of 88,000 miners, 20 per cent were HIV-positive, and 75 per cent of the 400–500 sex workers around it were HIV-positive as well.[19]

With more and more government officials contracting HIV, governance will become a sham in South Africa. It is reported that in South Africa as many as one in seven civil servants are

[12] Ibid, p. 5.

[13] Ibid.

[14] Ibid.

[15] 'HIV/AIDS as a Security Issue', ICG Report, p. 9.

[16] 'South Africa's Ambassador Sisulu Defends Her Government's AIDS Policy: Addresses anti-PhRMA demonstration in the United States', 12 March 2001, available at http://www.globaltreatmentaccess.org/content/press_releases/a01/031201_WF_HGAP_phrma.html.

[17] Price-Smith, 'Pretoria's Shadow', p. 13.

[18] Ibid.

[19] Elbe, 'Strategic implications of HIV/AIDS', p. 48.

thought to have been HIV-positive in 1998.[20] The disease is also selectively targeting skilled workers, middle and senior management, educated urban professionals and government officials.[21] While health workers are supposed to be in the know of the ways and means of avoiding infection, it has been reported that in a survey conducted in 2003 '16 per cent of 2000 surveyed health workers were HIV-positive, with at least 20 per cent of those aged 20 to 35, living with the virus'.[22] The education sector is in an equally pathetic shape. As many as a third of the teachers are HIV positive and 5 die daily due to the illness.[23] The fact that in a 1999 survey '[a]t the University of Durban-Westville in Kwazulu-Natal, 25 per cent of the student body recently tested positive for HIV', shows that the best talents in the country are going to fall prey to HIV/AIDS in the years to come.[24]

In South Africa, AIDS permeates the police and the military to such an extent that they are not permitted to donate blood.[25] Reports say that not even 50 per cent of the South African National Defence Force is combat ready for a variety of reasons including high rates of HIV/AIDS infection in it. Many officers, reportedly, are not willing to enter into combat situations along with soldiers who are HIV-positive as it may lead to exposure to HIV.[26] A report in 2004 claimed that 'an overwhelming 89 per cent of those soldiers who volunteered for testing were HIV-positive'.[27]

[20] 'The Destabilising Impact of HIV/AIDS', CSIS, 2002.

[21] 'HIV/AIDS as a National Security Issue', ICG Report, p. 100.

[22] Dr Chinua Akukwe, 'HIV/AIDS in Africa: South Africa's Leadership is Crucial', 14 August 2003, available at http://www.theperspective.org/aids_southafrica.html.

[23] Ibid, p. 16.

[24] Alex Kirby, 'South Africa's growing HIV crisis', 7 June 1999, available at http://news.bbc.co.uk/1/hi/sci/tech/363232.stm.

[25] Ibid.

[26] Price-Smith, 'Pretoria's Shadow', p. 21.

[27] The report further said that 1,089 soldiers had volunteered to be tested, of whom 947 were found to be HIV-positive. The average age of the sample was 34, and 60 per cent of volunteers were married. '89% South African Military HIV/AIDS Shocker', *The Independent Online* (*IOL*), Cape Town, 12 August 2004, available at http://www.rense.com/general56/sdhock.htm.

The country's Defence Minister Mosiuoa Lekota has gone on record saying that 17 per cent of the 70,000-strong South African military is HIV-positive.[28] As a result, many of these infected forces are unable to participate in international peacekeeping operations.[29]

Within the South African police force also, the rate of HIV is on the increase. Over 33,000 of the 1,35,000 police forces are now confirmed HIV-positive. This, according to both the South African Police Union and the Police and Prison Civil Rights Union, will lead to serious shortages in trained personnel in the police forces.[30]

Why is South Africa where it is today? The AIDS Review 2000, released in April by the Centre for the Study of AIDS at the University of Pretoria and written by Hein Marais, points out some very important reasons for this.[31] First, due to the mismanagement of the AIDS control programme in the country, people became bored, dismissive and fatalistic. Second, the untimely restructuring of the public health sector hampered the implementation of the government's AIDS programme which consistently underspent on its budget. Third, there was a complete lack of consultation in the government's AIDS campaign, along with a tendency towards centralized decision-making and a 'siege mentality.' The result has been that as well as the relevant non-governmental players, even the department's own HIV/AIDS and sexually transmitted diseases directorate was left out of the consultative loop. Finally, the number of scandals related to the AIDS-control programme distracted both the public and the politicians from the AIDS epidemic itself and polarized those important stakeholders who should have been allies in the fight against HIV/AIDS.

Jo Stein, Principal Scientific Officer at the AIDS and Society

[28] Price-Smith, 'Pretoria's Shadow', p. 18.

[29] Ibid., p. 22.

[30] Ibid, p. 4.

[31] Jo Stein, 'Chances lost in the war on AIDS: Review tells a sorry tale of contradictory policy decisions', Urban Health And Development Bulletin, vol. 3, no. 2, June 2000. Available at http://www.mrc.ac.za/urbanbulletin/june2000/lostchanges.htm.

Research Unit of the Centre for Social Research at the University of Cape Town, notes that HIV-prevalence in both Thailand and South Africa was less than 1 per cent in 1990, and eight years later it was 1.5 per cent in Thailand compared to over 22 per cent in South Africa.[32] What made the difference in the case of Thailand? Can countries like India learn something from the Thai experience?

THAILAND'S SUCCESS STORY

From epidemic proportions to unbelievable lows through proactive committed anti-AIDS programmes, that is the Thai story of how it confronted the deadly disease. While the first AIDS case was reported in Thailand in 1984, the disease hit the public imagination in 1988–9 when 'HIV-infection exploded among injecting drug-users, rising from almost nil to 40 per cent in a single year. At almost the same time, a second wave of infection spread among sex workers. In 1989, it was found that 44 per cent of sex workers in Chiang Mai, in the north, were infected with HIV. The rising infection level among sex workers launched subsequent waves of the epidemic in the male clients of sex workers, their wives and partners, and their children.'[33] In 1991, there were 1,42,819 new infections which were reduced to 23,676 by 2002.[34] How was this made possible? It is necessary to look at the ways and means adopted by the Thai government to combat the infection as it shows how single-minded and result-oriented programmes can bear fruit in the long run.

Since most of the country's infections resulted from its rampant commercial sex, the country's main focus was to ensure 100 per cent condom use in the country. The following steps were taken in order to reduce the infection rates in the country.

- 100 per cent condom use in brothels

[32] Ibid.

[33] Annabel Kanabus and Jenni Fredriksson 'HIV and AIDS in Thailand', available at http://www.avert.org/aidsthai.htm.

[34] 'Asian Nations Lag In War On AIDS', 30 November 2003, available at http://www.cbsnews.com/stories/2003/11/30/health/main586011.shtml.

- Mass advertising campaigns promoting condoms during commercial sex
- Free condom distribution by the government
- Emphasis on workplace education on HIV/AIDS
- Testing and treating and condom distribution to individual sex workers through routine exams
- Getting reports from male sexually transmitted infections (STI) patients leading to more outreach
- Regular visits of health workers for prevention, testing and treatment
- Establishment of mobile clinics
- Strong political and financial commitment at local and national levels
- A social worker with NGO experience chosen to head the programmes and report directly to the prime minister
- Strict controls imposed on brothels which were asked to implement 100 per cent condom use failing which they would be shut down[35]
- More condom-vending machines in public places[36]
- Every schwas required to conduct AIDS education classes.[37]

On the one hand, while compulsory one-minute AIDS prevention ads were broadcast on TV and radio every hour, in several communities, Buddhist monks taught villagers about condom use and how the disease is spread and preached the need to accept AIDS sufferers. The temples went on to host support groups, and a hospice where monks specialized in preparing herbal medicine that alleviates symptoms was set up.[38] One of the important aspects of the anti-HIV/AIDS programme of Thailand was that everyone in the country was involved in it in some way or the other. 'Every segment of Thai society played a role in AIDS prevention. Everyone from the medical community to teachers,

[35] Kim Ciabattari, 'HIV success: The 100% condom program in Thailand', available at www.fic.nih.gov/dcpp/ppts/padian.ppt.

[36] Kanabus and Fredriksson 'HIV and AIDS in Thailand'.

[37] Ibid.

[38] 'Asian Nations Lag In War On AIDS', 30 November 2003.

to monks, to prostitutes and to drug addicts was part of the programme. The government committed funds for research and backed private organizations that attempted to spread the word about how to stop AIDS. Even the powerful Thai military pitched in, running voluntary blood tests for soldiers.'[39] While it was a perfectly directed campaign, it was not just a top-down approach; grass-roots community activism was given great importance in the entire process.[40]

CONCLUSION

This chapter has argued that the experiences of most African countries in dealing with HIV/AIDS have been neither easy nor successful. The deadly disease has eaten into almost all sections of those countries: military, police, society, education, family structure etc. The South African example shows us how not taking care of the disease can be catastrophic. The Thai experience of dealing with the disease shows us that well-planned and mass-based programmes can reverse the pace and the spread of the disease.

[39] Kanabus and Fredriksson 'HIV and AIDS in Thailand'.

[40] Simon Montlake, 'Asia looks to Thailand's AIDS success story', 20 November 2003, *Christian Science Monitor.*

CHAPTER 5

Conclusion: Where are We Heading?

The basic argument that this study has made is that security, as Barry Buzan says, is a sectoral concept and not a monolithic one as people have traditionally perceived it. Moreover, this sectorization need not be done in a predefined manner; sectors of security or, in other words, dimensions of security, can be formulated keeping in mind the spatio-temporal context.

It also suggests that there need not be a 'single-referent-object' of security. While state-centric security discourses have emphasized the state as the referent object of security, anthropocentric views of the universe would have the human person as the ultimate referent object of security. This study suggests that what the referent object of security is can be decided only after analysing the spatio-temporal context of the threat in question. The attempt here is not to give security a 'comprehensive nature'; rather, it is about identifying the referent objects of security in a given context.

HIV/AIDS has been viewed as a security threat from this perspective. The paper has argued that the deadly disease is a threat to India's state, individuals, society, and economy. The referent object(s) of security here are those that are threatened by the disease: the state, individuals, society, and the economy.

The first chapter has argued that HIV/AIDS will prove to be a security threat to India given the fact that it is rapidly spreading to the general population and rural areas of the country, which is compounded by the fact that there are claims and counterclaims about the extent of HIV/AIDS-infection in the country. Even an intermediate figure between the highest and the lowest claims would mean that there are around 7 to 8 million infections in the country. Factors such as homosexuality and infected blood transfusion only exacerbate the problem. The chapter concludes with an argument that the future scenario of HIV/AIDS in the country is likely to be disturbing due to, first, the high mobility of the population, second, the nature of the population that is getting infected—young and dynamic—third, the rampant poverty in the country which will translate into increased sex work for subsistence reasons and diminished chances for getting adequate health care, and fourth, the size of the population which will hobble attempts to highlight the issue to the larger public.

The second chapter has made the following arguments: first, HIV/AIDS destroys human security at both individual and collective levels by way of causing individual suffering and death, causing the HIV/AIDS victims to contract other opportunistic diseases, fall prey to the normal Indian practice of treating the victims social outcasts, and killing people at an extremely productive and reproductive age; second, despite the lack of any comprehensive data regarding the exact nature of the economic losses to the country due to HIV/AIDS, available figures have suggested that the HIV/AIDS-related economic burden can be huge.

Moreover, HIV/AIDS can also slow down the flow of foreign direct investment into India, create problems for India's foreign trade, affect household economy and savings, put additional budget and other burdens on the health sector which is already in bad shape, and deprive non-HIV-infected people going to hospitals of treatment. The disease can also adversely affect sectors such as IT, tourism, and transportation. HIV/AIDS can also impact, the paper argues, India's bilateral relations, it's peacekeeping operations abroad and policing within the country.

Further, India's societal security can also be jeopardized by HIV/AIDS. AIDS orphans may eventually become social outcasts who would then turn to anti-social activities; social institutions like the family and marriage could lose their sanctity; and regional discords and distrusts could eventually develop as the epidemic spreads far and wide.

The third chapter argues that HIV/AIDS can prove to be extremely dangerous in a country like India when combined with poverty which is still very extensive, ignorance about the disease which is not uncommon in many parts of India where the epidemic seems to be growing, and the stigma associated with the disease. While even one of these factors can make HIV/AIDS deadly in its pace of growth, all three factors in tandem are seen to increase the incidence of the disease.

While malnutrition and lack of health care decrease the chances of survival of those who are HIV-positive, poverty prompts people to take to professions like sex work which increases the incidence of HIV/AIDS. The poor also tend to sell their blood to earn a living: this blood, which is often contaminated, can increase the incidence of the disease.

It was argued that ignorance can make HIV/AIDS deadlier due to three reasons: first, nine out of ten people infected do not know they are HIV-positive and are likely to go on spreading it; second, those not infected are not aware of the disease and may engage in risky behaviour; and third, the general public, due to the lack of knowledge may not accept HIV/AIDS prevention programmes as is increasingly been seen in many parts of the country. Stigma, the paper argues, contributes to the suffering of those infected and their relatives, interferes with decision making on HIV counselling and testing for HIV status, and seeking and remaining with prolonged treatment.

The final chapter has argued that the experiences of most African countries in dealing with HIV/AIDS have been neither easy nor successful. HIV/AIDS has affected almost all sectors of those countries: military, police, society, education, family structure, etc. The South African example is illustrative in this regard. The Thai experience of dealing with the disease shows us that well-planned and mass-based programmes can reverse the pace of the spread of the disease.

The burden of this paper, for the most part, was to demonstrate that HIV/AIDS is proving to be a security threat to India in a variety of ways. The mandate of this paper is not to suggest ways and means to contain the problem on which considerable research is already underway. However, it would be appropriate to point out some important areas of focus with regard to the HIV/AIDS crisis in the country. The following aspects are crucial and thus need to be kept in mind while making HIV/AIDS-related policies:

- While it is true that Indians are afflicted by many serious diseases equally or more deadly HIV/AIDS, due to its peculiar nature, needs to be given a very important place in the country's health-care system.
- In India, religions mostly turn a blind eye towards HIV/AIDS or prevent its followers from adopting family planning methods like condom usage as in the case of Catholics. Religions need to wake up to the urgency of the situation and call upon its followers to actively engage in anti-AIDS campaigns. Priests of all religions should be urged to take the lead in this respect.
- Like terrorism and war, HIV/AIDS too needs to be accorded the status of a security issue as according a special status invariably means allocation of more funds and special consideration, etc.
- There is an acute need to set up anti-AIDS cells in the industrial centres of the country, including factories, business enterprises, IT industry, call centres, etc.
- There has to be a comprehensive programme covering India's main transportation arteries to drastically reduce the spread of the disease as transportation is one of the most important means by which rural India is getting infected by HIV/AIDS. The ongoing efforts are no more than minimal.
- India needs to shed its complacent thinking on the issue of HIV/AIDS, that as a country it is doing enough; India is a huge country and thus tiny measures will not help.
- It is time the Indian government changed its archaic thinking on sex work and sexual minorities. The government should legalize both so that the disease, can be addressed more openly and confronted more successfully.
- Public opinion and public imagination in India can do wonders. Political parties need to instruct their cadres to take up the issue of HIV/AIDS and create awareness among the people. India needs charismatic leaders to address the issue.
- India needs to have a more sensible AIDS-surveillance programme which includes rural areas, private health sectors, etc., so that people know where they stand.
- In a country like India, where grass-roots policies and Panchayati Raj institutions have traditionally played a commendable role,

albeit not in the entire country, such institutions and movements need to be mobilized to address the issue.

- India has much to learn a lot from the Thai experience, including:
  1. Getting religions to talk openly about the issues relating to HIV/AIDS,
  2. Setting up condom-vending machines in badly affected areas, and
  3. Putting compulsory advertising on HIV/AIDS on TV every hour.
- Last but not the least, it would be advisable for the country to have a very experienced person in the HIV/AIDS sector with the rank of a minister in the Union Cabinet or the Prime Minister's Office to coordinate HIV/AIDS-related activities in the country. He/she need not be under the Ministry of Health, but should report directly to the prime minister.

Bibliography

'AIDS and the military: UNAIDS point of view, May 1998, available at www.worldbank.org/wbi/aidsleadership/ dls_AIDS_military_may14.pdf.

'AIDS cases up by 610,000', *Business Standard*, New Delhi, 14 November 2003.

'AIDS control program in Bihar a total failure', *Times of India*, New Delhi, 15 July 2001.

'AIDS explosion alert', *The Telegraph*, Calcutta, 2 March 2001.

'AIDS in India', 26 June 2001, online interview appeared in *The NewsHour*, available at http://www.pbs.org/newshour/bb/health/jan-june01/aidsindia_6-26.html

'AIDS spells faster death in India than in US, says study', *Indian Express*, New Delhi, 27 December 2001.

Akukwe, Chinua, 'HIV/AIDS in Africa: South Africa's Leadership is Crucial', 14 August 2003, available at http://www.theperspective.org/aids_southafrica.html.

'Alarm over AIDS on India-Nepal border', *Agence France Press*, 23 August 2000, available at http://w3.whosea.org/healthnews/ie24aug.htm.

'Alarming increase in HIV/AIDS cases in Bihar', *Hindustan Times*, New Delhi, 9 March 2002.

Anand, K., C.S. Pandav, L.M. Nath, 'Impact of HIV/AIDS on the National Economy of India', *Health Policy*, vol. 47, no. 3, June 1999.

'Asian Nations Lag In War On AIDS', 30 November 2003, available at http://www.cbsnews.com/stories/2003/11/30/health/main586011.shtml.

'At-A-Glance–India: AIDS and orphans', Vasavya Mahila Mandli, available at http://www1.worldbank.org/sp/safetynets/OVCWorkshop_5-03/Handout_ India.pdf.

Bajpai, Kanti, 'Human Security: Concept and Measurement', Kroc Institute Occasional Paper, August 2000, available at http://www.nd.edu/~krocinst/ocpapers/op_19_1.PDF.

Beyrer, Chris, 'Accelerating and Disseminating Across Asia', *The Washington Quarterly*, Winter 2001, available at http://www.twq.com/winter01/beyrer.pdf.

Bharat, Shalini, 'India: HIV and AIDS-related Discrimination, Stigmatization and Denial', August 2001, available at www.thebody.com/unaids/pdfs/india.pdf.

Bharat, Thiyam, 'HIV/AIDS and Socio-Economy', 8 July 2002, available at http://www.manipuronline.com/Features/July2002/hivandsocioeconomy08_1.htm.

Booth, Ken, 'Security and Emancipation' *Review of International Studies*, vol. 17, 1991.

Boxer, Barbara, 'Providing Basic Human Security', *The Washington Quarterly*, Spring 2003, available at www.twq.com/03spring/docs/03spring_boxer.pdf.

Buzan, Barry, *People, States and Fear: An Agenda for International Security Studies in the Post-Cold War Era*, Boulder: Lynne Reinner Co., 1991.

Carter, Michael, 'Sexual transmission of HCV seen in Indian women with genital ulcers and men who have sex with men', 30 July 2003, available at http://www.aidsmap.com/news/newsdisplay2.asp?newsId=2217.

Chaudhuri, Mohuya, 'Indian Migrant Workers: Sweatshop conditions/ignorance lead to AIDS epidemic', available at http://www.comminit.com/Commentary/sld-4103.html.

Ciabattari, Kim, 'HIV success: The 100% condom program in Thailand', available at www.fic.nih.gov/dcpp/ppts/padian.ppt.

Claxton, Isabelle, 'The right to know', *Seminar*, 520, December 2002.

Cowley, Geoffrey, 'A deadly passage to India', *Newsweek*, New York, 25 November 2002, available at http://www.blackherbals.com/a_deadly_passage_to_india.htm.

Derian, James Der, 'The Value of Security: Hobbes, Marx, Nietzsche, and Baudrillard,' in Ronnie Lipschutz (ed.), *On Security*, New York: Columbia University Press, 1995.

Eberstadt, Nicholas, 'The Future of AIDS', *Foreign Affairs*, November/December 2002.

'Economic costs of AIDS', World Bank Group, 23 July 2003, available at http://www.globalpolicy.org/socecon/develop/2003/0723costs.htm.

'89% South African Military HIV/AIDS Shocker', *The Independent Online (IOL)*, Cape Town, 12 August 2004, available at http://www.rense.com/general56/sdhock.htm.

Ekstrand, Maria, Lisa Garbus, Elliot Marseille, 'HIV/AIDS in India', AIDS Policy Research Center, University of California San Francisco, August 2003, p. 6, available at http://ari.ucsf.edu/ARI/policy/profiles/India.pdf.

Elbe, Stefan, 'Strategic implications of HIV/AIDS', *Adelphi Paper*, no. 357.

Gannon, John C., Chairman, NIC, 'The Global Infectious Diseases Threat and its Implications for the United States', January 2000, available at http://www.cia.gov/cia/reports/nie/report/nie99-17d.html.

Gilks, C, 'Impact on the Health system in India', summaries of publications from UNDP Asia-Pacific Regional Project on HIV and Development, available at http://www.hivundp.apdip.net/Regional/Publication%20The%20 Economics%20of%20AIDS.pdf.

Gorden, David F., 'The Next Wave of HIV/AIDS: Nigeria, Ethiopia, Russia, India, and China', US Intelligence Community Assessment, September 2002, p. 1, available at www.cia.gov/nic/PDF_GIF_otherprod/HIVAIDS/ICA_HIVAIDS20092302.pdf.

Gordon, Peter, Ruth Jacobson and Tom Porteous, 'A Study to Establish the Connections Between Hiv/Aids & Conflict', February 2004, available at http://www.jsiuk.com/docs/hiv_aids_conflict_2004.pdf.

'Growth of AIDS in India declines', The New Delhi Television, 6 July 2004 (New Delhi), available at http://www.ndtv.com/template/template.asp?id =56707&template=AIDS&callid=1&frmsrch=1&txtsrch=hiv%2Faids.

Gupta, Indrani, 'Do we still need more evidence?' *Seminar*, 520, December 2002.

Gupta, Indrani, Samiran Panda and Renuka Motihar, 'HIV/AIDS and Development in India', Background Study for the Swedish Country Strategy for India 2003–2007, February 2003, available at www.countryanalyticwork.net-CAW-Cawdoclib.nsf-vewWhatsnew Latest Document-33E1C61C8AE8E58885256E31004D8FF6-$file-HIV-AIDSD.

Gupta, Kamla and S.K. Singh, 'Social Networking, Knowledge of HIV/AIDS and Risk-Taking Behaviour among Migrant Workers', p. 8, available at http://www.iussp.org/Bangkok2002/S06Gupta.pdf.

Gupta, Rajan, 'HIV/AIDS poses a threat to India: A global perspective', available at http://t8web.lanl.gov/people/rajan/AIDS-india/MYWORK/issues.9.99.html.

'HIV positive soldier challenges dismissal in court', 26 October 2003, *Agence France-Presse*. Accessed at http://www.aegis.com/news/afp/2003/AF031095.html.

'HIV prevention: Should there be compulsory screening?', *BBC Online*, 29 November 2002, available at http://news.bbc.co.uk/1/hi/talking_point/debates/south_asian/2511103.stm.

'HIV/AIDS as a Security Issue', ICG report, p. 3, available at www.crisisweb.org/home/getfile.cfm?id=510&type=pdf.

'HIV/AIDS as a Security Issue', International Crisis Group, 19 June 2001, available at http://www.crisisweb.org//library/documents/report_archive/A400321_19062001.pdf.

'HIV/AIDS in India', http://www.genetics.wayne.edu/asg/hivindia.html.

'HIV/AIDS in South Africa', http://www.avert.org/aidssouthafrica.htm.

'India faces explosion in HIV/Aids', 14 August 2004, available at http://www.guardian.co.uk/india/story/0,12559,1282852,00.html.

'India to have 110 million HIV/AIDS victims by 2025', 25 August 2004, available at http://www.newindpress.com/Newsitems.asp?ID=IEH20030708132100&Title=Top+Stories&rLink=0.

Italia, Y.M., I.S. Gilada, ' Invisible Entry of HIV in Rural India, Visibly Distort India's Socioeconomic Fabric', XIV International Conference on AIDS, Barcelona, 7-12 July 2002, available at http://www.iaen.org/files.cgi/7035_italia.pdf.

Iype, George, 'No Longer Mecca for Prosperity'. 7 July 2004, available at http://specials.rediff.com/news/2004/jul/07spec.htm.

Jayasekera, Deepal, 'AIDS becomes a serious health problem in India', 4 May 2001, available at http://www.wsws.org/articles/2001/may2001/aids-m04.shtml.

Joseph, Josy, 'Indo-US defense cooperation on HIV/AIDS program', 11 March 2004, available at www.rediff.com.

'K'taka intends law for compulsory HIV test before wedding', *Hindustan Times*, New Delhi, 2 August 2004, available at http://www.hindustantimes.com/2004/Aug/02/181_924562,000900020002.htm.

Kanabus, Annabel and Jenni Fredriksson, 'HIV and AIDS in Thailand', available at http://www.avert.org/aidsthai.htm.

Kirby, Alex, 'South Africa's growing HIV crisis', 7 June 1999, available at http://news.bbc.co.uk/1/hi/sci/tech/363232.stm.

Lisk, Franklyn, 'Labour Market and Employment Implications of HIV/AIDS', June 2002, ILO Programme on HIV/AIDS and the World of Work, Geneva, June 2002, available at www.ilo.ru/aids/docs/wp/wp1_labourmarket.pdf

Mahal, Ajay, 'Economic implications of inertia on HIV/AIDS and Benefits of Action', *Economic and Political Weekly*, 6 March 2004.

McPherson, Malcolm, 'The Macroeconomic Impact of HIV/AIDS', available at www.iris.umd.edu/ppc_IDEAS/HIV_AIDS/01_29_03.asp.

McPherson, Malcolm, Deborah Hoover, and Donald Snodgrass, 'The Impact on Economic Growth in Africa of Rising Costs and Labor Productivity Losses Associated with HIV/AIDS,' Working Paper, Kennedy School of Government, Harvard University, 2000, available at http://www.cid.harvard.edu/caer2/htm/content/papers/bns/dp79bn.htm.

Menon, Subhadra, 'India's Widening AIDS Epidemic', *BBC Online*, 28 November 2003, available at http://news.bbc.co.uk/2/hi/south_asia/3250285.stm.

Montlake, Simon, 'Asia Looks to Thailand's AIDS Success Story', 20 November 2003, *Christian Science Monitor.*

'Mumbai police face mandatory HIV testing', 28 January 2004, www.worldvision.org/worldvision/pr.nsf/stable/update_india_012804.

Mutimer, David, 'Beyond Strategy', in Craig A. Snyder (ed.), *Contemporary Security and Strategy*, London: Macmillan, 1999.

NACO, National Baseline General Population Behavioural Surveillance Survey, conducted by NACO: New Delhi, 2001, available at http://www.naco.nic.in/nacp/publctn.htm.

Nandakumar, Prathima, 'Vadodara has 6,000 HIV positive cases', *Times of India*, New Delhi, 17 May 2003.

National AIDS Control Organisation, http://www.naco.nic.in/indianscene/esthiv.htm.

'National Family Health Survey (NFHS-2), 1998–99: India', available at www.nfhsindia.org/data/india/indintro.pdf.

Ninan, Ann, 'Without my consent: Women and HIV-related stigma in India', available at www.prb.org/Template.cfm?Section=PRB&template=/ContentManagement/ContentDisplay.cfm&ContentID=8278.

'Number of HIV-infected women growing in UP', *Times of India*, New Delhi, 28 March 2001.

'One crore Indians may be affected by AIDS', *Times of India*, New Delhi, 13 May 2001.

'1 per cent of pregnant women are HIV positive', *The Pioneer*, New Delhi, 2 November 2001.

'1800 Railway employees have AIDS and 200 Railway Employees have died of AIDS', *India Today Online*, May 2003.

Palanigounder, Duraisamy, 'Economic impact of HIV/AIDS on patients and households in South India: costs and burden on households and coping strategies', available at www.iaen.org/ files.cgi/9838_EcoImpact-HIV-AIDS-SouthIndia.doc.

Panigrahy, Sisir, 'AIDS spurt in Orissa district raises alarm', *Indian Express*, New Delhi, 15 January 2002.

Price-Smith, Andrew, 'Pretoria's Shadow: The HIV/AIDS pandemic and national security in South Africa', 2002, p. 7, available at http://www.cbaci.org/specialreport4pricesmith.pdf.

Project Memorandum written by the Department of International Development (DFID), London, in 1996, available at http://www. unescap.org/tctd/pubs/hiv01_2_6.htm.

'Punjab minister calls migrants a health threat', *Indian Express*, New Delhi, 4 December 2001.

Sambamoorthi, Usha et al., 'Antenatal care and AIDS knowledge among married women', *Economic and Political Weekly*, 14 February 2004.

Sarkar, Sudeeshna, 'Nepalese workers contracting HIV in India: Report', *Hindustan Times Online*, New Delhi, 19 August 2003.

Schaffer, Teresita C., Pramit Mitra, 'India at the crossroads: Confronting the HIV/AIDS Challenge, A Report of the CSIS HIV/AIDS Delegation to India', 3–10 January 2004, p. 10, available at www.csis.org/saprog/0401_ hivindia.pdf

Schneider, Mark, Michael Moodie, 'The destabilizing impacts of HIV/AIDS', May 2002, available at http://www.csis.org/africa/0205_DestImp.pdf.

'7 Madurai School kids test HIV-positive', *Indian Express*, New Delhi, 31 January 2003.

Shah, Nitin, 'HIV/AIDS', http://www.medivisionindia.com/aids/index.phtml.

Sharma, Rohit, 'More than a quarter of India's youngsters have pre-marital sex', *British Medical Journal*, 10 March 2001, available at http://bmj.bmjjournals.com/cgi/content/full/322/7286/575.

Singh, Pawanpreet, '30 labourers return with AIDS', *Times of India*, New Delhi, 20 March 2004.

Solomon, Suniti, Aylur Kailasm Ganesh, 'HIV in India', International AIDS Society – USA, *Topics in DIV Medicine*, vol. 10, no. 3 July-August 2002, p. 20, available at http://www.iasusa.org/pub/topics/2002/issue3/july_august 2002.pdf.

'South Africa's Ambassador Sisulu Defends Her Government's AIDS Policy: Addresses anti-PhRMA demonstration in the United States', 12 March 2001, available at http://www.globaltreatmentaccess.org/content/press_releases/a01/031201_WF_HGAP_phrma.html.

Srivastava, Arun, 'AIDS unknown to sex workers in Gaya: Study', *Indian Express*, New Delhi, 21 May 2001.

Stein, Jo, 'Chances lost in the war on AIDS: Review tells a sorry tale of contradictory policy decisions', *Urban Health And Development Bulletin*, vol. 3, no. 2, June 2000, available at http://www.mrc.ac.za/urbanbulletin/june2000/lostchances.htm.

'Summary Report: Behavioural Surveillance Survey in Healthy Highway Project, India: Part 4', Family Health International, 2001, available at http://www.fhi.org/en/HIVAIDS/pub/survreports/BSSHealthyHwy/BSSHealthyHwy4.htm.

'The HIV/AIDS crisis in India', *South Asia Monitor*, Centre for Strategic and International Studies, 1 May 2003, available at http://www.csis.org/saprog/sam58.pdf.

'10 per cent of AIDS affected are children', *Hindustan Times*, New Delhi, 6 November 2001.

'Terrorists spreading AIDS in J&K', *Daily Excelsior*, Jammu, 31 March 2004, available at http://www.dailyexcelsior.com/web1/04mar31/news.htm.

Terzieff, Juliette, 'AIDS prevention workers say police harass them as crisis spirals', *San Francisco Chronicle*, San Francisco, 17 November 2002, available at http://www.aegis.com/news/ads/2002/AD022240.html

'UN Says India May Overtake South Africa in AIDS Cases', 5 June 2002, available at http://www.hivandhepatitis.com/recent/developing/050602f.html.

'Use of infected Indian blood. 16 border Dists. at risk of HIV/AIDS', 6 August 2002, www.nation-online.com.

Varma, Mitu, 'India–Health: AIDS Watch, Poverty Watch', 26 September 1997, available at http://www.aegis.com/news/ips/1997/IP970908.html.

Verma, Ravi K. et al., 'HIV/AIDS and children in the Sangli district of Maharastra', in Giovanni Andrea Cornia, *AIDS, Public Policy and Child Well-Being*, available at http://www.unicef-icdc.org/research/ESP/aids/chapter8.pdf.

'Women are becoming increasingly affected by HIV', *The Pioneer*, New Delhi, 8 March 2002.

'World Population Prospects: The 2002 Revision', p. 85, available at www.un.org/esa/population/publications/wpp2002/wpp2002annextables.pdf.

RCSS PUBLICATIONS

- *Defence, Technology and Cooperative Security in South Asia: Report on the Proceedings of the Tenth Summer Workshop* (RCSS, 2004)
- *Environment Development and Human Security: Perspectives from South Asia* (2003)
- *Terrorism in South Asia: Impact on Development and Democratic Process* (SIPRA, 2003)
- *South Asia and the War on Terrorism* (India Research Press, 2003)
- *Shaping the Future–A South Asian Civil Society Dialogue* (RCSS, July 2002)
- *Small Arms and Human Insecurity* (RCSS, July 2002)
- *SAARC in the Twenty-First Century: Towards a Cooperative Future* (July 2002)
- *Memories of a Genocidal Partition: The Haunting Tale of Victims, Witnesses and Perpetrators* (RCSS, July 2002)
- *South Asian Security Futures: A Dialogue of Director's Regional Strategic Studies Institutes* (March 2002)
- *Security and Governance in South Asia* (September 2001)
- *Globalization and Non-Traditional Security in South Asia* (September 2001)
- *Security in the New Millennium* (India Research Press, 2001)
- *The Simla Agreement 1972: Its Wasted Promise* (Manohar, 2001)

RCSS Newsletter

A quarterly bulletin, it publishes a brief report of RCSS activities, presentations at its workshops on topics of contemporary interest and news and programmes of the RCSS and its alumnae.

RCSS Policy Studies

35 Nuclear Risk Reduction Measures in South Asia: Problems and Prospects (Manohar, 2005)
34 Indo-Pak Conflicts: Ripe to Resolve? (Manohar, 2005)
33 Small Arms and the Security Debate in South Asia (Manohar, 2005)
32 New Nuclear Triangle and China's Role in South Asia (2005)
31 Stability through Economic Cooperation in a Nuclear Environment (Manohar, 2005)
30 Multi-Track Diplomacy between India and Pakistan: A Conceptual Framework for Sustainable Security (Manohar, 2005)
29 The Role of Mediation in Resolving India-Pakistan Conflict: Parameters and Possibilities (Manohar, 2005)
28 HIV/AIDS as a Security Threat to India (Manohar, 2005)
27 Nepal's Maoist Movement and Implications for India and China (Manohar, 2005)
26 Elite Perceptions in Foreign Policy: Role of Print Media in Influencing India-Pakistan Relations, 1989-1999 (Manohar, 2004)
25 Nuclear Risk Reduction Measures and Restraint Regime in South Asia (Manohar, 2004)
24 River Water Sharing Problem Between India and Pakistan: Case Study of the Indus Basin Water Treaty (June 2004)
23 Christianity and Political Conflict in India: The Case of Gujarat (June 2002)

Fellowship in South Asian Alternatives (FISAA) Monograph

- Water, Power and People: A South Asian Manifesto on the Politics and Knowledge of Water (1997)
- The Nuclear Debate: Ironies and Immoralities (1998)

Others

- *Directory of Individuals and Institutions Engaged in South Asian Strategic Studies* (1998).

Rov Blatt